Community Based Rehabilitation

. . . it is more important to bring about even small improvements among masses, than to provide the highest standard of care for a privileged few. (B. O'Toole (1990) In: Practical Approaches to Childhood Disability in Developing Countries: Insights from Experience and Research, Thorburn, J. J. and Mario, K. (Eds), pp. 293–316. Memorial University of Canada, Newfoundland.)

The evolution of CBR worldwide as an integral component of primary health care reveals political and moral commitment to achieve equal opportunity and social integration for disabled persons. We have no choice but to succeed; at essence is the dignity of each of us. (G. Chermak (1990) International Disabilities Studies **12**(3): 123–127.)

Community Based Rehabilitation

Malcolm Peat MCSP, DipTP, MPT(Manitoba),
MSc(Manitoba), PhD(Manitoba)
Executive Director
International Centre for the Advancement of
Community Based Rehabilitation, Queen's University,
Kingston, Ontario, Canada

WB Saunders Company Ltd
London   Philadelphia   Toronto   Sydney   Tokyo

WB Saunders Company Ltd
24–28 Oval Road
London NW1 7DX, UK

The Curtis Center
Independence Square West
Philadelphia, PA 19106–3399, USA

Harcourt Brace & Company
55 Horner Avenue
Toronto, Ontario M8Z 4X6, Canada

Harcourt Brace & Company, Australia
30–52 Smidmore Street
Marrickville, NSW 2204, Australia

Harcourt Brace & Company, Japan
Ichibancho Central Building, 22–1 Ichibancho
Chiyoda-ku, Tokyo 102, Japan

A catalogue record for this book is available from the British Library

ISBN 0-7020-1941-0

Typeset by J&L Composition Ltd, Filey, North Yorkshire
Printed and bound in Great Britain by The Bath Press, Bath, UK

Contents

Preface   ix
Acknowledgements   xi

**Chapter 1: Introduction to
    Community Based Rehabilitation**   1

**Chapter 2: The Magnitude of
    Disability**   4
Definitions of Disability   4
Demographics of Disability   6
Disability in More Developed
    Regions   10
Disability in Less Developed Regions   11
Types of Disabilities   14

Chapter 3: Community   16
Introduction – What is Community?   16
Community Defined   16
Multiplicity of Communities   20
The Community Based Approach   20
Community Entry Strategies   21
Community Based Rehabilitation
    and Community Development   22
Community Initiated versus
    Community Oriented   22
Community Participation and
    Mobilization   23

**Chapter 4: Community Based
    Rehabilitation**   27
Introduction to Community Based
    Rehabilitation   27

Historical Review   28
Defining the Concept of
    Community Based Rehabilitation   30
The Changing Ideology of
    Community Based Rehabilitation
    – a Spirit of Tolerance   31
Composition of Community Based
    Rehabilitation   31
Strengths and Weaknesses of
    Community Based Rehabilitation   34
A Descriptive Framework of
    Community Based Rehabilitation   34
The Continuum   36
Community Based Rehabilitation
    Strategy   37
The Community Oriented Approach
    to Rehabilitation   38
Service Strategies for Community
    Based Rehabilitation   39
Service Coordination   41
Community Based Vocational
    Rehabilitation and the
    International Labour Organization   41
Strategies for Changes toward
    Community Based Rehabilitation   42
Professional and Bureaucratic
    Challenges   43
Community Based Rehabilitation in
    Areas of Conflict   44

Chapter 5: Community Based Rehabilitation Models 48

Defining and Classifying CBR Models 48

Models of CBR 49

Chapter 6: Planning and Management of Community Based Rehabilitation Programmes 72

Introduction 72

CBR Programme Planning and Management 72

Ownership and Governance 73

Decentralization and Community Based Rehabilitation 74

Management of Community Based Rehabilitation Programmes 74

Programme Sustainability 85

Communication and Coordination 86

Community Participation, Mobilization and Awareness 88

CBR Programme Influence on Promoting and Developing Public Policies 89

Chapter 7: Evaluation in Community Based Rehabilitation 90

Introduction 90

What, How and Why to Evaluate 90

Quantitative versus Qualitative Data 94

Uses of Evaluation Findings 94

Participatory Evaluation 95

Models of Evaluation 95

Chapter 8: Education in Community Based Rehabilitation 98

Community Based Rehabilitation Knowledge Base 98

Transfer of Knowledge and Skill 99

Stakeholders in the Educational Process 99

Strategies in Education 101

Critical Factors in the Design and Implementation of CBR Educational Programmes 102

Potential Problems in CBR Training Programmes 103

Educational Systems in CBR 104

Chapter 9: The Economic and Social Consequences of Disability, and the Organization of Persons with Disabilities 113

Introduction 113

Economics of Disability 114

What is Empowerment? 119

Charitable Organizations 122

Organizations of Persons with Disabilities 122

Uni-disability and Cross-Disability Organizations 129

The Consumer Movement 129

Role of Women 131

Chapter 10: Research in Community Based Rehabilitation 135

Introduction 135

Who is Interested in Research? 136

The Goal of Research in Community Based Rehabilitation 136

Difficulties in CBR Research 137

CBR Research Topics 138

Partnerships in Research 141

Research in Less Developed Countries 142

Chapter 11: Policies, Strategies and Services 143

Introduction 143

Making Policy 143

Public Participation in the Development of Policy 144

Strategic Planning Process and Public Policy Development 146

Government Policies 149

Non-government Organization Policies 150

Multilateral International Development, Government and Non-government Collaborative Policies 150

A Brief Comparison of Government and Non-government Organizations 151

Human Rights Policy 151

Chapter 12: Conclusion   156
Deciding the Future   156
Challenges to the Current System   157
The Objective of Community
   Based Rehabilitation   158

Flexibility in Approach   158
Demonstrating the Value of
   Community Based Rehabilitation   159

Index   161

Preface

Who is the Book For?

Community based rehabilitation (CBR) has become a major feature of the design of programmes for persons with disabilities and a core element in the restructuring of health and social programmes in both industrialized and developing societies. This book is written primarily for those involved in the application of CBR and in the education of the key stakeholders in the CBR process, including professionals in the health and social sciences, non-government and government agencies, consumer groups and community organizations.

What is the Book About?

The book is intended to be a basic text which examines the development of CBR and the factors influencing its design and implementation. CBR is discussed in relationship to the uniqueness of communities and the needs of persons with disabilities. CBR is viewed as part of a continuum ranging from the person with a disability in the community to the specialized regional rehabilitation facility. The factors influencing the development of CBR, which include planning, management, education, research, evaluation and policy issues, are viewed with the perspective that there is no single approach that represents CBR.

Why was it Written?

The author has been involved in the development of services and educational programmes and has participated internationally in the development of CBR, working with government agencies, non-government organizations, universities and consumer groups. The text is based on the experience of working with, and learning from, persons with a disability. As CBR is a relatively new and innovative approach, information on its diversity and application is limited. The text provides a review of both the formal and informal literature on the subject, and is intended for a broad audience.

Malcolm Peat

Acknowledgements

The author would like to acknowledge the community of persons with disabilities and colleagues in organizations for persons with disabilities for their guidance and influence in enhancing the author's understanding of disability and quality of life issues and for their invaluable advice.

I would also like to express my sincere appreciation to the members of the International Centre for the Advancement of Community Based Rehabilitation and its international partners and colleages at Queen's University for their cooperation and collaboration. In particular, I would like to recognize Lorna Jean Edmonds for her generous personal support and constructive advice throughout the production of this work.

Early in the development of this text I was assisted by Jenana Jalovcic, Verla Fortier, and through the development of the book, I received the editorial advice of Enid Peat. This book would not have been completed, however, without the exceptional contribution made by Carolyn Pinkerton through editing and developing text and concepts.

Introduction to Community Based Rehabilitation

To rehabilitate, from its original Latin meaning, is to restore not to create. Terms such as 'restoration' 'reinstatement' 'redevelopment' and 'return to normal' have been used more recently to define the term rehabilitation. In the legal and medical literature, rehabilitation refers to a process of restoring to a former capacity by focusing on residual and recoverable functions and capacities. In the development of health, social and community programmes, it has been difficult to arrive at one precise definition for the term rehabilitation that effectively represents the interests and needs of persons with disabilities, their families and communities, while at the same time articulating the understanding of the academically and clinically based health professional. As a result, neither the disabled person nor the public or health professionals have reached a consensus about what needs to be done, what can be done, and who can provide the services (Matkin, 1985).

It has been suggested that the aim of rehabilitation has been misunderstood and its methods misapplied. These problems reflect a lack of coordination between professional groups from which rehabilitation has borrowed its technology including medicine, surgery, biomechanics, psychology, education and sociology. Rehabilitation has, in effect, undergone three overlapping phases in its development:

♦ the pioneering phase – characterized by flexibility;
♦ the status phase – characterized by rigidity and adherence to rules and regulations;
♦ the expansion phase – characterized by tolerance (Peat, 1981).

The Ontario Ministry of Health (OMH), Canada in 1995 provided the following definition of rehabilitation:

Rehabilitation is a progressive, dynamic goal-oriented and often time-limited process which enables an individual with an impairment to identify and reach his or her optimal mental, physical, cognitive, and/or social functional level. Rehabilitation provides opportunities for the individual, the family and the community to accommodate a limitation or loss of function and aims to facilitate social integration and independence. (OMH, 1995)

Another view is that rehabilitation is a process which combines interventions focused on the person with disabilities, plus environmental modifications and adaptations to achieve a successful rehabilitation outcome. How an individual views rehabilitation depends upon personal experience, including one's social and political view of disability issues.

♦ *Consumers and their families*, and *advocates* who may be expecting, demanding or receiving services might view rehabilitation as everything a person with a disability requires to live an independent and productive life.
♦ *Health and social professionals and other service providers* might see rehabilitation in terms of what can reasonably be provided, given financial constraints and the priorities driving the system.
♦ *Funders* of rehabilitation services may view it with fairly rigid or defined boundaries in order to limit or control expenditures within identified national priorities.
♦ *Designers and planners* of rehabilitation services may take a more expansive view of the definition in order to ensure that all necessary connections to other systems are facilitated.
♦ *Regulators of services* might define rehabilitation in terms of those distinct provider groups or activities or identifiable individuals that can be monitored (OMH, 1995).

In the past 25 years, rehabilitation services, like other aspects of Western health care, have been concentrated in specialized institutions. The *'medical model'* for health care and rehabilitation emphasizes predominantly urban-based, medical specialist institutional care. While this significantly advanced the scientific and research base of professional practice, it left observable shortfalls in the development and implementation of accessible and user-friendly programmes. The pressure for the expansion and development of services for the person with a disability is not the result of one factor, but a number of related issues such as decreasing resources, increasing demands, increasing population and limited health manpower (Peat and Boyce, 1993).

Community based rehabilitation (CBR) has emerged as a primary contender in the search for a practical and successful means of providing appropriate health care to a greater percentage of the disabled population. 'The major objectives of community based rehabilitation are to ensure that persons with disabilities are able to maximize their physical and mental abilities, have access to regular services and opportunities and achieve full social integration within their communities and societies. These objectives are developed from the broader concept of rehabilitation which includes equalization of opportunities and community integration' (ILO, UNESCO, WHO, 1994).

CBR is recognized as a comprehensive approach which encompasses disability prevention, rehabilitation in primary health care activities, integration of disabled children in ordinary schools and provision of opportunities for gainful, economic activities for disabled persons (ILO, UNESCO, WHO, 1994). As a component of social policy, CBR promotes the rights of individuals to live within their communities and participate fully in its economic, social, political and cultural life. CBR is appropriate and applicable to both economically advantaged industrialized societies and developing, economically challenged regions.

Internationally, the rehabilitation services sector consists of a complex array of public and private programmes and services. While all involved stakeholders agree on the importance of CBR, there is some concern that it has no clear central approach – there are as many varieties of approaches as there are CBR programmes. In some societies CBR was seen as a 'grassroots' rural development strategy and not applicable to the urban environment. There are, however, many successful CBR programmes in both urban and rural regions and in both economically advantaged and disadvantaged societies, which supports the concept that there is no one absolute strategy, or any one group with ownership over CBR. Throughout the development of CBR in the last twenty years, there has been debate, dissension and even rivalry between the differing perspectives and approaches. It is unfortunate that a great deal of the literature debates institutional versus community based services and assumes that they are mutually exclusive. CBR has a place as does institutional practice in the rehabilitation continuum.

CBR must be seen by the person with disability, the family and community, health professionals and society in general as *belonging to the community*. It should be considered a critical component of social, educational and health policy at national, regional and community levels. *CBR needs to be part of a country's action plan for all disabled persons* (WHO, UNESCO, ILO, 1994).

This text discusses CBR by appreciating the diversity of communities in which it occurs and the alternative strategies available. The text also reviews the magnitude of the problem of disability, policy issues, management practices, education and research, and emphasizes the necessity of involving persons with a disability in all aspects and levels of CBR and the need for all participants in the process to appreciate that CBR is primarily a partnership.

REFERENCES

International Labour Organization (ILO), United Nations Educational, Scientific and Cultural Organization (UNESCO), World Health Organization (WHO), (1994) *Joint Position Paper on Community Based Rehabilitation for and with People with Disabilities*, Geneva.

Matkin, R. E. (1985) Rehabilitation: an ambiguous term and an unfulfilled ideal. *Rehabilitation Literature* **46**(11–12): 314–320.

Ontario Ministry of Health (1995) *Ontario Rehabilitation Services Strategy*. Toronto, Canada.

Peat, M. (1981) Physical therapy: art or science. *Physiotherapy Canada* **33**(3): 170–176.

Peat, M. and Boyce, W. (1993) Canadian community rehabilitation services: Challenges for the future. *Canadian Journal of Rehabilitation* **6**(4): 281–289.

chapter
two

The Magnitude of Disability

DEFINITIONS OF DISABILITY

Several important trends are influencing the development of rehabilitation and the understanding of disability issues. Major social, economic, political and technological changes have shaped the future of persons with disability and handicap and facilitated the restructuring of services for disabled persons and their families (Symington, 1994).

The major trends shaping the understanding of disability issues are:

♦ the changing demography of disability and handicap;
♦ the emancipation of persons with disability;
♦ the policy shift from isolation to integration of persons with disabilities;
♦ the increasing costs of health and social services;
♦ the shift from institution based to community based programmes (Naisbett and Aburdeen, 1990).

The International Classification of Impairments, Disabilities and Handicaps

The *International Classification of Impairments, Disabilities and Handicaps* was published by the World Health Organization in 1980 (Figure 2.1). These definitions improved communication and understanding and introduced a framework that enhanced policy formulation, data collection, statistical analysis and the exchange of information.

The definitions of disability proposed by the World Health Organization have gained wide acceptance. This classification has reduced the confusion that was caused by the often interchangeable use of the terms: *impairment, disability, handicap* (Figure 2.1).

In simple terms, disability is defined as any reduction in the ability to perform activities in a manner which is normal, while handicap describes the social disadvantages resulting from an impairment or a disability. There are a number of ways that disabilities can be more specifically defined. One approach is to define

WHO Classification of Impairments, Disabilities and Handicaps.

Impairment is any loss or abnormality of psychological, physiological, or anatomical structure or function. It is characterized by losses or abnormalities that may be temporary or permanent, and that include the existence or occurrence of an anomaly, defect, or loss of limb, organ, tissue, or other structure of the body, including the systems of mental function. Impairment represents exteriorization of a pathological state, and in principle it reflects disturbances at the level of the organ. It represents deviation from some norm in the individual's biomedical status, for example, the loss of a limb.

Disability is any restriction or lack (resulting from an impairment) of ability to perform an activity in the manner, or within the range, considered normal for a human being. Disability is characterized by excess or deficiencies of customarily expected activity, performance and behaviour, and these may be temporary or permanent, reversible or irreversible, and progressive or regressive. Disabilites may arise as a direct consequence of impairment or as a response by the individual, particularly psychologically, to a physical, sensory, or other impairment. Disability represents objectification of an impairment, and as such it reflects disturbance at the level of the person. Disability is concerned with abilities, in the form of composite activities and behaviours, that are generally accepted as essential components of everyday life. Examples include disturbances in behaving in an appropriate manner, in personal care (such as excretory control and ability to wash and feed oneself), in the performance of other activities of daily living, and in locomotor activities, for example, the inability to walk.

Handicap is a disadvantage for a given individual, resulting from an impairment or a disability, that limits or prevents the fulfilment of a role that is normal (depending on age, sex, and social and cultural factors) for that individual. Handicap is concerned with the value attached to an individual's situation or experience when it departs from the norm. It is characterized by a difference between the individual's performance or status and the expectations of the individual himself or of the particular group of which he or she is a member. Handicap thus represents socialization of an impairment or disability, and as such it reflects the consequences for the individual – cultural, social, economic and environmental – that stems from the presence of impairment and disability. Handicap thus occurs when there is interference with the ability to sustain what might be designated as 'survival roles', for example, the inability to work because one's office is on the fifth floor of a building without an elevator.

Figure 2.1

disability according to function. Functional limitations and/or activity restrictions can make a person with a disability physically, psychologically or economically dependent on the person's family or community. Functional activities include moving, seeing, speaking and hearing.

It has been suggested that these definitions are most appropriate to a medical based approach to rehabilitation and that a more socially appropriate definition needs to be considered. The disability movement, led by Disabled Peoples' International (DPI), has played a crucial role in introducing definitions of impairments and disability that favour the social, as opposed to the medical, model (Figure 2.2). DPI argues that in practice there is no difference between 'loss of function' (impairment) and the 'lack of ability to perform' (disability).

Disabled Peoples' International Classification (Figure 2.2)

At present, definitions of disability vary in the emphasis they place on the role of the environment as a contributing factor to handicap. For example, when a loss is the physical loss of a limb, there is a tendency to define the disability according to the loss of movement. Definitions that include the influence of social factors have been proposed placing the loss of the limb in a social context. Disability is the loss of a limb, and the effect of this loss on function.

When defining disability and handicap, the economic, social and physical environments must be taken into consideration (Figure 2.3). The economic environment comprises the opportunities for employment, integration and independence and the extent to which these are possible for the person with a disability. The social environment is influenced by the beliefs, attitudes and behaviours that surround a person with a disability, that are communicated to him or her as positive or negative impressions. The physical environment includes the natural and architectural structures that affect the person with a disability, and limit or promote physical activities. The economic, social and physical environments play an important role in transforming an impairment into a disability. Variations between cultures therefore affect both the meaning of disability and the environment in which persons with disabilities live.

The recent focus on disablement, which is defined as the process leading to disability and handicap, has fostered the development of techniques to measure the process and its impact. Several theoretical models of the disablement process are listed below.

◆ *Biomedical Model* – focusing on pathology and physical change.
◆ *International Classification of Disability and Handicap Model* – disability, handicap, impairment.
◆ *Situational Handicap Model* – how disability affects function in different life situations.
◆ *Quality of Life Model* – how disability influences acceptance, family life and social interaction (Minaire, 1992).

DEMOGRAPHICS OF DISABILITY

The global prevalence of moderate to severe disabilities is estimated to be

Disabled Peoples' International Classification of Impairment and Disability

An *impairment* is the loss or abnormality plus the effect on function.

A *disability* is the disadvantage or restriction of activity caused by social factors which take little or no account of people who have impairments and thus exclude them from the mainstream of social activities.

(DPI, 1990).

Figure 2.2

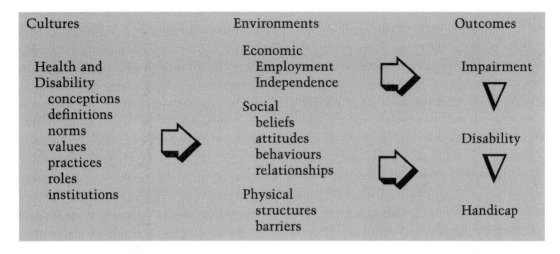

Figure 2.3 The role of the economic, social and physical environment in transforming an impairment into a disability (Berry and Dalal, 1996).

Table 2.1 Global estimate of prevalence of severe and moderate disability (Helander, 1993)

Based on United Nations population projection 1990	More developed regions	Less developed regions	Total
Total population (millions)	1207	4086	5293
Prevalence of moderate and severe disability (%)	7.73	4.47	5.21
Number of persons with moderate and severe disability (millions)	93.3	182.2	275.5

about 5% in less developed regions and about 8% in more developed regions (Table 2.1). Disability has emerged as a major health and social problem worldwide, common to countries with wide-ranging levels of socioeconomic development. Seventy-five per cent of the world's population, 86% of all babies born, and 98% of all childhood deaths occur in less developed regions (Figure 2.4). One billion people live in poverty with a life expectancy of less than 50 years. One-third of the world's disabled are children and two-thirds suffer from preventable disabilities. Eighty per cent of the world's disabled persons live in isolated rural areas in developing regions. Large numbers of these lack access to preventive, curative or rehabilitative services.

Interpretation of Disability Statistics

The interpretation of disability statistics is complicated and should be viewed with caution. Developed regions have proportionately more people with disabilities than less developed regions. This discrepancy may be explained by variations in attitudes to disability, survey mechanisms, the presence of health and social services and the age composition of the population.

Age

In addition to cultural variations in identifying and reporting disability, the age

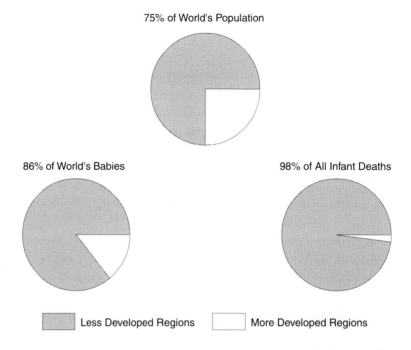

Figure 2.4   Infant mortality in less developed and more developed regions (Noble, 1981).

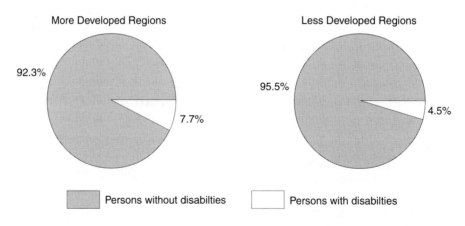

Figure 2.5   Comparison of percentage of population with disabilities in more developed and less developed regions (Noble, 1981).

composition of a population is a large factor contributing to the discrepancy in the prevalence rate between more developed and less developed regions (Figure 2.5). In general, the incidence of disability increases with age. More developed countries have more senior citizens per capita. In demographic terms, the global estimate of disability is 'age dependent'.

Reporting Mechanisms

There are few reliable demographic studies of less developed regions as reporting methods are not standardized and are often too expensive to be implemented effectively. Identification of people with disabilities in less developed regions of the world is often accomplished through questionnaires, and rarely by direct physical examination and observation.

The costs of national surveys are high and undertaking surveys is often a low priority both administratively and financially. In some instances where persons with disabilities are invited to participate in disability surveys, they have done so with the expectation that rehabilitation and other services would follow and often this has not occurred. When developing survey instruments, it is important to obtain estimates using socially, as well as demographically, appropriate methods. Accurate data collection on the magnitude of disability is still a problem, given that in some societies disability is identified by diagnostic category (e.g., spinal cord injury) and in others by classification of the loss of function (e.g., cannot walk). Drawing comparisons between these two categories would be inappropriate. A major challenge for policy-makers and governments is to standardize disability data collection in a way that is cost efficient and accurate, as well as socially and culturally acceptable.

The demographic, economic and social factors in developed and less developed regions influence the disability profile and the statistical differences reported. Two issues that complicate the interpretation of global disability numbers are the identification of disability and the definition of disability. Several global estimates of the prevalence of disability have been made in the last twenty years. The WHO 1976 data estimated that 10% of the world population was disabled. Since that time a number of studies have been completed. However, the results show a great variation in the prevalence of disability. For example, a study in China in 1987 showed 4.8% as the prevalence rate (Cochrane, 1983). The differences can be attributed to different survey methods and the inclusion criteria used.

Trends in Population and Factors that Influence Disability:

In more developed regions
♦ Sickness and injury (morbidity) rate is increasing.
♦ Death rate is decreasing (mortality).
♦ Disability rate is increasing faster than the population rate.

In less developed countries
♦ Population is increasing exponentially.
♦ Death rate is expected to decrease.
♦ Sickness and injury rate is expected to increase.
♦ Disability rate is increasing faster than the population rate.

In global terms
♦ Population rate is increasing exponentially.
♦ Death rate is decreasing.
♦ Sickness and injury rate is increasing.
♦ Disability rate is increasing (Naisbett and Aburdeen, 1990).

Poverty and Disability

Poverty and disability are inextricably linked in all societies. A person with a disability is more likely to experience poverty and impoverished regions have greater difficulty in addressing the economic and social needs of disabled persons and their families. Poverty is more than just a lack of income; it also is a lack of influence, power, information and resources and control over basic life decisions.

♦ *Relative poverty* is when people are poor in relation to the average standard of living in their country and when they lack the goods and services needed to live a fulfilling life in that society.

♦ *Absolute poverty* is when people are so poor that they lack enough of the basic goods and services needed to live at a minimum standard.

Persons living in poverty are at risk of becoming disabled because of:

♦ a lack of food or balanced diet;
♦ unhealthy and unsafe living environment;
♦ low-paid, dangerous and insecure employment;
♦ exposure to violence;
♦ a lack of access to health facilities and treatment;
♦ high illiteracy rate, lower education level which prevents access to information (Tiroler, 1992).

DISABILITY IN MORE DEVELOPED REGIONS

A number of factors influence the changing pattern of disability in developed regions. For example, in the 1930s and 1940s tuberculosis and poliomyelitis were the predominant causes of disability. The advent of antibiotics and vaccines, and the implementation of preventive measures, resulted in a significant reduction in these disability-producing diseases. Trauma is an increasing cause of disability in North America (Symington, 1994). For example, the incidence of spinal cord injury and traumatic brain injury is on the increase. Since 1950, the range of physical disabilities considered appropriate for physical rehabilitation has expanded and includes arthritis, soft tissue injuries, stroke, and cardiac and pulmonary disorders.

Based on a health and disability survey in Canada in 1983–4 (Statistics Canada, 1986), the prevalence of various disability groups in Ontario was estimated as:

♦ Developmental disabilities   79 344
♦ Visual   119 000
♦ Hearing   237 000
♦ Mental illness   264 480
♦ Disability resulting from
     restricted mobility   622 000
Total (= 15% of the total
     population)   1 321 824

While the causes of disability have been changing, other factors also influence the demographic profile including the ageing of the population and the increasing life-span of individuals with a disability.

The Ageing of the Population

Arthritis, cardiovascular and respiratory diseases are primarily diseases of the elderly. The general population in Western society is ageing, increasing the incidence of disability significantly. One in ten of North America's population today is 65 or older. Within 25 years, this figure will rise to one in five. More than 25% of patients surveyed who were seen by family physicians were over 65 (Almind et al., 1985) and a British study showed that 60% of disabled persons were over 65 (Cochrane, 1983). Most surveys on the incidence of disability and ageing agree that the incidence of disability increases sharply with age.

In terms of prevalence and cost, disability ranks as North America's largest health problem. Developed regions have more seniors per capita than less developed regions. It is estimated that 85% of Americans now over the age of 65 are living vital and active lives and many work by choice, explore new opportunities, and meet new challenges (Symington, 1994). However, the chance of becoming disabled increases significantly after the age of 80.

The Increasing Lifespan of Individuals with a Disability

Disabled persons are living longer and with ageing, disability tends to increase. Disabled younger persons are beginning to outlive their primary caregivers, creating an additional demand on the rehabilitation system. Advances in technology and improvements in emergency responses and facilities have increased the number of persons surviving life-threatening events such as trauma and neonatal emergencies. Also, statistics show that there is an increase in the number of persons with multiple disabilities. The survival of those with severe disability, although relatively small in number, places a heavy demand on rehabilitation resources (Symington, 1994).

Twenty-five per cent of North Americans live in towns with a population of 2500 or less. The concentration of rehabilitation resources in urban areas means that disabled persons living in rural areas have less opportunity to make use of the wide range of rehabilitation resources that are available (Cook and Ferritor, 1985). Only 15% of disabled persons in rural areas of the United States get professional help and the situation in Britain appears to be somewhat the same. Gloag (1985) stated that there was a vast amount of unmet need in rehabilitation in Britain. It is perhaps surprising to learn that the pattern of underutilization of services in developing regions is also apparent in North America. The low utilization of services is particularly noticeable in societies where there is a difference in expectations and cultural orientation

between service providers and clients. In Western society, the pool of health professionals is drawn from the middle classes with low representation by minority groups and the immigrant population.

DISABILITY IN LESS DEVELOPED REGIONS

Most of the world's population live in less developed regions and it has been estimated that rehabilitation services are reaching no more than 2% of the total disabled population in these regions (WHO, 1981). It has been suggested that the situation has not significantly changed since the 1960s and 1970s. In a comprehensive survey representing 33 countries with half the world's population, James (1984) estimated there to be 14 million physically handicapped persons, of whom one in six needed some form of special device. However, only 1% had any form of assistance whatsoever.

One reason for the unchanging situation is that many less developed regions have adopted professional roles and services which may be inappropriate to the needs and structure of their societies. The development of rehabilitation in the last twenty years has been influenced by the perception that Western skills, knowledge and attitudes in rehabilitation practice should be adopted by developing societies. This problem is compounded by the shortage of health professionals in the area of rehabilitation with little possibility that the current manpower supply will ever meet the demands of the disabled population in less developed societies.

Rehabilitation services in less developed regions are influenced by:

- over-concentration of services on an urban elite;
- the adoption of unnecessarily high

standards of training for rehabilitation professionals;
- the narrowness of specialization;
- unnecessary confinement of persons with disabilities to institutions;
- unnecessary unemployment (O'Toole, 1987; Symington, 1994).

In developing societies, each year over 3 million children die and 3 million are disabled. An estimated two-thirds of these disabled children have disabilities that are vaccine preventable (Figure 2.6).

With current efforts to improve health care in less developed regions, it is expected that:

- disability prevention measures will result in a decrease in communicable diseases and malnutrition;
- the expected survival rate will continue to increase quite considerably;
- increased urbanization, more traffic, more industrial development, deterioration of water and sanitation systems are likely to contribute to increased incidence of disability;
- better education and health care, lower pregnancy rate, improved housing, shorter working hours and better communications may decrease the occurrence or severity of disability (Noble, 1981).

However, it is believed that the positive effects of prevention will be more than offset by the increased survival rate of those over 65 years in less developed countries. By the year 2025, the number of senior citizens over 65 years of age living in less developed regions will increase 212% (Table 2.2).

The largest population growth will be in the over 30 age group. As a result the age profile of less developed regions will begin to resemble that of the more developed regions of the world.

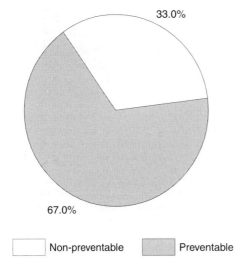

Figure 2.6 Preventable childhood disabilities in less developed regions (Noble, 1981).

Global Estimates of Disability

By the year 2025, there will be at least 435 million people in less developed regions

Table 2.2 Population in less developed regions projected by age group (Helander, 1993)

Age group	Population in millions		Growth (%)
	1990	2025	
0–4	544	620	+14
5–14	909	1225	+35
15–29	1178	1782	+51
30–64	1273	2955	+132
65+	182	568	+212
Total	4086	7150	+75

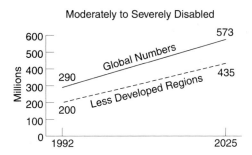

Figure 2.7 Global estimate of disability in developed regions (UNDP, 1993).

with moderate to severe disabilities, or more than twice the current number (Figure 2.7). The rate of global disability is increasing rapidly, mostly due to population growth and population ageing in less developed regions (Figure 2.8).

Globally four major factors contribute to disability:

+ congenital or perinatal (birth) disturbances – 18%;
+ communicable diseases – 23%;

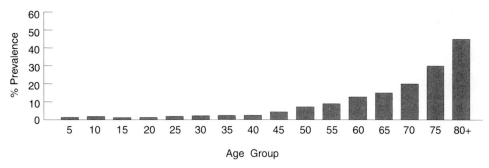

Figure 2.8 Global prevalence of disability by age group (UNDP, 1993).

Table 2.3 Global causes of disability and prevalence of moderate and severe disabilities (UN Statistical Office, 1990; Helander, 1993)

Causes of disability	Global estimates of the prevalence of severe and moderate disabilities expressed in millions (world population 5300 million)
Congenital or perinatal disturbances	
Mental retardation	10–20
Somatic hereditary defects	10–25
Non-genetic disorders	15–20
Communicable diseases	
Poliomyelitis	5–10
Trachoma	8–10
Leprosy	3–4
Other communicable diseases	30–40
Non-communicable somatic diseases	70–80
Functional psychiatric disturbances	15–20
Alcoholism and drug abuse	25–30
Trauma/Injury	
Traffic accidents	15–20
Occupational accidents	10–12
Home accidents	15–20
Other	2–3
Malnutrition	7–10
Other	2–3
Estimated total	250–300

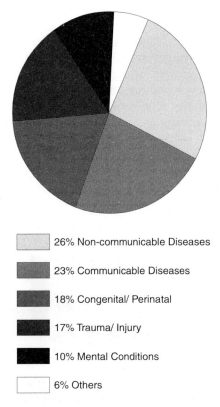

26% Non-communicable Diseases

23% Communicable Diseases

18% Congenital/ Perinatal

17% Trauma/ Injury

10% Mental Conditions

6% Others

Figure 2.9   Global causes of disability (Helander, 1993).

♦   non-communicable somatic (physical) and mental conditions – 36%;
♦   trauma and injury – 17%.

A description of what is referred to under the heading 'communicable diseases' is included in Table 2.3.

TYPES OF DISABILITIES

In less developed regions the most commonly identified disabilities are related to loss of, or interference with, mobility. Following this, hearing, speech, and vision are the identified categories. In Canada, in 1982, mobility was identified as the largest category, followed by mental illness, hearing, vision and developmental disorders. Figure 2.10 compares types of disability in Canada and Indonesia.

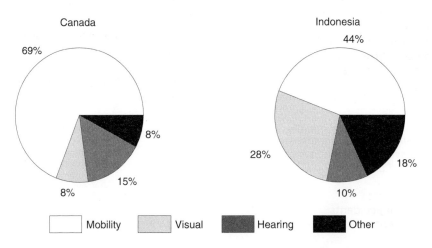

Figure 2.10   Comparison of types of disability in Canada and Indonesia (Johnson and Tjandraksuma, 1982).

REFERENCES

Almind, G., Freer C., Gray, J. and Warshaw, G. (1985) The contribution of the primary care doctor to the medical care of the elderly in the community. *Danish Medical Bulletin* **32**(2): 1–28.

Berry, J. and Dalal, A. (1996) *Disability, Attitudes, Beliefs and Behaviours. Report on an International Project in Community Based Rehabilitation*. ICACBR, Queen's University, Kingston, Canada.

Cochrane, G. M. (1983) Aids in the home. *British Journal of Hospital Medicine* **29**: 121–126.

Cook, D. and Ferritor, D. (1985) The family: a potential resource for the provision of rehabilitation services. *Journal of Applied Counselling and Development* **55**(2): 15–16.

Disabled Peoples' International (DPI) (1990) – *DPI Accomplishments Information Sheet*. Winnipeg, Manitoba.

Gloag, D. (1985) Severe disability: residential care and living in the community. *British Medical Journal* **290**: 369–371.

Helander, E. (1993) *Prejudice and Dignity. An Introduction to Community Based Rehabilitation*. United Nations Development Program, New York.

James, W. V. (1984) Technology for the disabled. *World Health Forum* **5**: 256–258.

Johnston, M. and Tjandraksuma, H. (1982) Reaching the disabled. *World Health Forum* **3**: 307–310.

Minaire, P. (1992) Disease, illness and health: theoretical models of the disablement process. *Bulletin of the World Health Organization* **70**(3): 373–379.

Naisbett, J. and Aburdeen, P. (1990) Megatrends 2000. In *New Directions for the 1990's*. William Morrow, New York.

Noble, J. H. (1981) Social inequity in the prevalence of disability. *Assignment Children* **53**(54): 23–32.

Ontario Ministry of Health, Ontario Ministry of Community and Social Services and Ontario Ministry of Citizenship, Government of Canada (1993) *Redirection of Long-term Care and Support Services in Ontario: A Public Consultation Paper*. Toronto, Queen's Printer for Ontario.

O'Toole, B. (1987) Community based rehabilitation (CBR): Problems and possibilities. *European Journal of Special Needs Education* **2**(3): 177–190.

Statistics Canada Health Division (1986) *Report of the Canadian Health and Disability Survey 1983–84*, Ottawa.

Symington, D. C. (1994). Megatrends in rehabilitation: a Canadian perspective. *International Journal of Rehabilitation Research* **17**: 1–14.

Tiroler, G. (1992) Learning about the Links. *CBR News AHRTAG*, No. 21, September/December, London.

United Nations Statistical Office (1990) *Disability Statistics Database and Compendium* (ST/ESA/Stat/Sery/2) (1976–86).

United Nations Development Program (UNDP) (1993) *Disabled People's Participation in Sustainable Human Development*. Division for Global and Interregional Programs.

World Health Organization (1981) *Global Strategy of Health For All by the Year 2000* (Health For All, Series 3) WHO, Geneva.

World Health Organization (1993) (1980) *International Classification of Impairments, Disabilities and Handicaps. A Guide for Development Agencies*. WHO, Geneva.

Community

INTRODUCTION – WHAT IS COMMUNITY?

This chapter reviews the concept of community. A precise definition of the term 'community' has long been a matter of sociological discussion and debate. Most of the literature agrees that a precise and single definition of the term 'community' may not be possible or indeed desirable.

The term community has many meanings and it has been used in many different ways. Community may mean a group of individuals who are *linked through common experiences*, philosophies, moral and social beliefs, prejudices and opinions. Community also exists as the social interaction among individuals who come together with the purpose of meeting needs or *organizing to achieve group goals*. Community in this sense is the collective action of individuals and is the sum of its organizations and institutions. Community is most commonly referred to as the *geographic* or *territorial* organization of people where they live and work (Poplin, 1972).

COMMUNITY DEFINED

For the purpose of reviewing community based rehabilitation, the following definition of community incorporates the elements of locality, organization and commonality:

A community consists of people living together in some form of social organization and cohesion. Its members share in varying degrees, political, economic, social and cultural characteristics, as well as interests and aspirations, including health. Communities vary widely in size and socio-economic profile, ranging from clusters of isolated homesteads to more organized villages, towns and city districts. (Helander, 1993)

Community as Locality

Definition (Oxford English Dictionary, 1975)

♦ Social interaction within a geographic area
♦ A population cluster
♦ A common location
♦ Living together in a place

The most common definition of community is the social and territorial locality of persons, in hamlets, villages, towns, cities and urban areas. This reference to community deals with the physical and spatial environment. It is the place in which people maintain themselves – where they work, make homes and generally carry out most of the activities of daily living (Poplin, 1972).

The community is a spatially limited area. Very often it is impossible to determine its exact boundaries, although they may have been arbitrarily established for political and governmental purposes. Because of constant changes within the community, establishment of rigid community boundaries could ignore its internal dynamics. Therefore the spatial area of the community is defined as a geographic area that contains social structures that meet the physical, psychological and social needs of the majority of its members. Many different geographical/environmental factors, such as topography, soil, cultivation, settlement pattern, and transportation system, influence the character of the community (Borkensha and Hodge, 1969). The environment in the geographical sense is an important factor that influences the needs of a particular community, and the needs depend on the characteristics of the environment.

In all communities there are critical resources that can be categorized as follows:

♦ *Human resources* of a community are professionals, laypersons, volunteers, citizens, including people with disabilities and their families. People are the single, most important resource for implementing any community based programme.
♦ *Physical resources* include buildings, equipment, services, supplies and natural resources occurring within the community such as private properties, municipal and local government structures, local service clubs holdings, resources of businesses and industries, and any tangible resources (other than personnel).
♦ *Structural resources* include municipal and other governments, local service club organizations, business and industry, institutions, religious orders, and any general community organization.

Community as Social Organization

Definition (Oxford English Dictionary, 1975)

♦ An interacting population of various kinds of mutually related individuals
♦ A group of people leading a common life according to a rule or discipline
♦ A group sharing particular economic, political, religious, linguistic or historical characteristics

Community in this sense means people linked by history, policies, politics, language or specific needs and implies the involvement of more than just one person. Traditionally the concept of community was associated with community spirit. The community can be viewed as a social activity marked by a feeling of unity in which individuals participate willingly and without losing their individuality or personal identity.

Leadership and Governance
Many successful community programmes have flourished as a result of exceptional leadership and commitment to a particular goal or set of objectives. All communities demonstrate structure and governance in the sense that the decision-making process must be apparent so that community members perceive themselves as participants in all aspects of

community decision-making. The concept of empowerment is the extent to which community members are fully involved in the life and organization of their environment. The governance structure of any community can range from a very complex, highly developed mechanism for decision-making to an informal sharing of ideas and concepts which permits a group to reach agreement or consensus through mutual support.

Historical Perspective

The experience of a community in dealing with major issues determines how a community may respond to issues and challenges. The historical perspective can be both a negative and a positive element in community development. The history of past events, both successes and failures, has a major influence on determining how a community will react to any new initiative. The historical perspective can also inhibit change where the community may be highly committed to a particular social, political or economic policy. The history of conflict very often renders a community unable to adapt and change through discussion and full community participation.

Existing Programmes

Most communities have some form of organized activity or existing programmes, and to some extent these are likely to be entrenched in community behaviour. Long established practice which may have led to the creation of vested interests can be an inhibiting factor in a community's ability to affect change. The perception of the public that rapid change is likely to occur can be threatening to a community as it can create uncertainty and insecurity. Successful community development can only occur where there is a balance between established practice and the

recognition of the need for constructive change.

Common Ties of Community

Definition (Oxford English Dictionary, 1975)

- Any group sharing interests and pursuits
- Persons who have one or more common ties
- People marked by common charateristics

The human community is not static, and should be approached as a dynamic condition. It can be viewed as a process involving social structure and cultural behaviour. This definition of community emphasizes common features, ties and interaction such as ethnic, racial, linguistic, religious or cultural dimensions (Borkensha and Hodge, 1969). Community members share various kinds of ties and bonds, ranging from kinship to common preferences. Communities consist of people in interaction with other people and with community systems, which forms a social network. The concept of the social network comprises all relationships of individuals among themselves, as well as their interaction with community groups and institutions. The type of social relations within community determines the choice of the community interventions that may be used (Borkensha and Hodge, 1969).

Many community programmes have developed as a result of the efforts and initiatives of a group sharing a common set of objectives. In many instances a community initiative has been a response to a lack of progress and the inability of the establishment to meet community needs. Many current community initiatives in both developing and developed regions are a result of a group of individuals acting on a common goal and objectives. For instance, advocacy groups representing the needs of the elderly population in North American and other societies have had a major influence on the development of health and social policies and the extent to which the political process can implement change.

Disadvantaged Groups in Communities

The needs and opinions of disadvantaged groups have often been ignored by society because of the unique cultural, political and power structure of society. Those who have power and control over wealth should guarantee the involvement of all groups in community life. Their voices must be heard especially in the planning and implementation of community based activities and the allocation of resources. This has often not been the case.

There are a number of communities which are recognized internationally as groups who are disadvantaged, through conflict, poverty, religion or ethnicity. There are also communities of refugees, the homeless and persons with disabilities who are denied equal and full participation in aspects of daily life. To establish a community, individuals must identify with a specific group and its members, and share common interests, preferences or needs. Identification of an individual with a community of persons with disabilities often depends on the concepts, beliefs and attitudes toward disability in society. The concept of disability varies significantly in different societies and very often has negative implications such as exclusion from many aspects of economic and social life.

A smaller community can give the feeling of security and belonging that society at large may not offer. Being set apart from the wider community, and identifying common problems and issues, has stimulated the formation of groups which focus, for example, on the special needs of women, the elderly and persons with disabilities. By exchanging their experiences these groups have realized that inaccessibility and exclusion are not problems unique to the individual, but rather they are societal problems, and through organized and common efforts, significant and positive changes can occur. By organizing themselves, disadvantaged groups can achieve a greater voice and more control over their own destinies and enhance participation in the decision-making process.

Family

Family structure is an important consideration in community life. The decision-making process for the family unit, the division of tasks and the appropriateness of participation may differ across cultures and ethnic groups. By supporting the family as a basic unit of the community, and by recognizing that certain individuals within the family structure may have specific needs, the community is strengthened.

Literacy/Poverty

Literacy affects not only one's ability to learn, but the methods of instruction and interaction. In community based rehabilitation (CBR) skill and information transfer is facilitated by a higher literacy rate. Disadvantaged groups such as women and persons with disabilities are particularly affected by poverty and have the highest illiteracy rates. Poverty is a variable which has a direct effect on programmes and priorities of community projects as it limits both the development of programmes and access to them.

MULTIPLICITY OF COMMUNITIES

In all societies an individual is often a member of several communities simultaneously. These can include communities related to religion, occupation, political affiliation, ethnicity, geographical location and gender. A person belongs to some communities because he or she has consciously chosen that community, such as a religious group or a group that forms around common characteristics such as language or tradition. Within all of these, there are many possible subsets of communities. For example, within one occupational group there can be a variety of levels of responsibility and decision-making. It is apparent that when an individual identifies with a particular community, he or she does so to address a particular need or set of circumstances. Individuals in the same family may share several common communities such as religion, ethnicity and socioeconomic status, but the individual family members may also belong to community groups to which the other family members do not subscribe, such as political, artistic or social associations.

An Individual as a Member of Many Communities.
The subject is a family woman, age 35, and a member of the community of:

♦ Canadians
♦ Francophones
♦ Nurses
♦ Mothers
♦ Immigrants
♦ Community Health Council
♦ Provincial College of Nurses
♦ Persons with a Disability
♦ Single Parents Association

Figure 3.1

Figure 3.1 is an invented example of an individual who is a member of various communities.

In this illustration, the person immigrated to Canada from Francophone Africa and was employed as a nurse in a French-speaking community in northern Manitoba, Canada. Following the dissolution of a marriage, she was responsible for a family of two daughters. As a nurse she has been very involved in the development of health programmes for minority groups and in this capacity is active politically in the local Community Health Council and the Provincial College of Nurses. As a result of an injury sustained while travelling, she is hearing impaired. In this social history, the individual can talk on behalf of many communities and participate in the development of all of them. This illustrates a situation that is common to many people which is that very few individuals are members of only one social or economic group or community.

THE COMMUNITY BASED APPROACH

The early 1970s was a period when this decentralized and participatory approach to programme planning and delivery gained popularity in many countries and in many areas of health and social development. The community based approach was developed in response to inefficient and centralized mechanisms for solving community problems. In community based programmes, the users of a service have some control over resources, from complete control to merely exerting a powerful influence (Bulmer *et al.*, 1989).

It has been suggested that most community based projects are specialized or functional agencies performing a clearly defined task, usually for a very specific population. The literature on community based programmes is extensive and includes public, commercial, charitable and voluntary activities. The development of community based rehabilitation is an example of an operation which impinges directly on the state and its social services (Bulmer *et al.*, 1989). In many instances CBR is the product of self-help groups, providing mutual support and care for members with a particular disability. In Britain in 1989, it was calculated that there were more than 1500 nationally organized disability related community groups nationwide with more than 25 000 regional branches. These included programmes related to cancer, heart disease, drug addiction, mental handicap, multiple sclerosis and many other disorders. In a comprehensive review of social policy and the development of community based programmes in Britain, Bulmer *et al.* (1989) stated that self-help groups providing the most comprehensive array of services, set an example which suggests the possibility of developing for a fairly clearly defined population, a broader community association capable of tackling any task the members want to turn their hands to'.

COMMUNITY ENTRY STRATEGIES

Entry into a community by individuals or groups must first involve an understanding and appreciation of the nature of the community including its diversity, organizations, boundaries, ties, interactions, and social and political frameworks. Imposition of a programme will likely lead to rejection and non-compliance. Ownership by a community is essential for successful sustainable programmes and implies understanding, participation and equality.

In the development of a community based rehabilitation programme in Bombay, successful entry into the community was obtained through a voluntary organization of women working with families in a heavily industrial and highly populated region of central Bombay. Although the local political and governance structures were all male dominated, this organization of women had gained respect and were trusted by the community for their work with residents to improve their quality of life. The women's group was well established and provided day-care, nutritional, and maternal and child health counselling services. A proposed rehabilitation programme was added to the existing initiative, and was introduced as a concept that focused on the needs of children with disabilities and their families. It provided support for the full integration of the children into community life including opportunities for education and recreation. The community, particularly the families of persons with disabilities, was involved in all aspects of the implementation and development process, and formed their own advocacy group. Rehabilitation programme activities were extended to include adults with disability within the community. This approach was successful as it was built on an existing and valued community programme which was organized, supported and maintained by the community. The sustainability of the programme focusing on persons with disabilities was assured by community acceptance and ownership of the programme, and the community assuming the responsibility for management and decision-making. The programme was also successful as it demonstrated partnership between health professionals from local agencies and the community, working with the mothers of the children with disability.

COMMUNITY BASED REHABILITATION AND COMMUNITY DEVELOPMENT

It has almost become a standard feature of modern political thought that the democratic process needs to be opened up to involve greater sectors of the population more directly in decision-making. Community participation in health and social programmes is considered to be central to all health and social development. Policy documents of international organizations and governments cite the importance of the need to engender community participation.

One of the common characteristics of CBR is that each CBR project is different. This difference has to be expected because CBR reflects the community where it exists, and communities are different. Differences are related not only to the uniqueness of communities, but to a variance in the ideology of those who initiate projects, differences that may prevent full community participation and ownership (Poplin, 1972).

Community Development
The United Nations definition of community development, in the context of community based rehabilitation, consists of programmes implemented to facilitate local communities, combining outside assistance with organized local self-determination and effort, so as to stimulate local initiative and leadership to change attitudes towards people with disabilities, and to assist people with disabilites with their development within their own community. (UNDP, 1991)

Community Based Rehabilitation
Community based rehabilitation is a strategy based on community development for the rehabilitation, equalization of opportunities and social integration of all people with disabilities themselves, their families and communities and the appropriate health, education, vocational and social services. Community based rehabilitation empowers persons with disabilities to take action to improve their own lives, and contribute rather than drain or deplete whatever scarce resources that are available, and thereby benefiting all the community. (ILO, UNESCO, WHO, 1994)

COMMUNITY INITIATED VERSUS COMMUNITY ORIENTED

When reviewing community programmes, it has to be understood that the term 'community' does not in itself imply ownership, participation or empowerment. Participation by the community is key to the success of any sustainable community development initiative. Community programmes can be either initiated within the community, or applied to it from an external source.

Community Initiated Projects
Very often a community based project starts without any external intervention, initiative or influence. These programmes are often referred to as 'grassroots' programmes which are developed in answer to a certain community need. The idea and concept of the project are conceived within the community with the main goal being to meet needs that have not been met by conventional means. These projects are governed and implemented by the community members who initiated the activities.

Community Oriented Projects

Community oriented programmes target a defined population of a community, and may involve its members in the implementation and decision-making process to a different degree. The most significant difference is that these programmes do not originate within that community. They are brought in from outside the targeted community and very often include external human and financial resources.

There are many activities related to health and social issues which are examples of community initiated and community oriented programmes. The critical element in both is the extent to which the community has a voice in programme development, direction and management.

COMMUNITY PARTICIPATION AND MOBILIZATION

'Community mobilization is the process of bringing together all intersectoral social allies to raise people's awareness of, and demand for, a particular development programme, to assist in the delivery of resources and to strengthen the participation of people to achieve project sustainability and self-reliance' (McKee, 1993). Successful programmes are those in which a community is truly distinguished by a set of shared interests. A community development programme depends on the mobilization and participation of those community members key to the theme of the programme. For example, maternal and child health programmes are of more relevance to women than to men. Hence, men would likely only be peripherally interested in the programme and therefore not necessarily part of the 'core' community.

Participation is key to all successful community development programmes. The *WHO Study Report on Community Involvement in Health* (1991) suggested that participation can be categorized in three ways:

♦ *participation as contribution* where the community participates through contributions including labour, financial resources, material products;
♦ *participation as organization* where the community creates appropriate structures to facilitate participation;
♦ *participation as empowerment* which involves groups and communities, particularly those who are poor and marginalized, developing the power to make real choices, and by having an effective voice and control.

It has also been suggested that community participation is a social process whereby specific groups with shared needs actively pursue the identification of their needs, make decisions, and establish mechanisms to meet these needs (Rifkin *et al.*, 1988). Community participation, however, will reflect local social and cultural values. Participation may not mean the same thing in different communities. Stone (1990) suggested that in Nepal community participation was promoted by the international organizations as self-reliance and equality. For the rural Nepalese, however, community participation was viewed as their contribution of land, labour or money. Consideration must be given to the structural and cultural issues at a community level when generating community involvement in health and social programmes.

Strengths of Community Participation

♦ More can be accomplished.
♦ Services may be provided at a lower cost.

♦ Participation has an intrinsic value for participants, alleviating feelings of alienation and powerlessness.
♦ Participation is a catalyst for further development efforts.
♦ Participation leads to a sense of responsibility for the project and eventual sustainability.
♦ Participation guarantees that people's needs are considered.
♦ Participation ensures the use of indigenous knowledge and expertise.
♦ Participation brings freedom from dependence on professionals.
♦ Participation helps people understand and question the nature of the constraints which are hindering their escape from poverty.
♦ Participation ensures that things are done the right way (McKee, 1993).

Barriers to Community Participation

♦ Participation may become ritualistic.
♦ Participation often depends on one charismatic leader.
♦ Participation may lead to the development of a participatory elite.
♦ Participatory experiments are often not cost-effective or replicable.
♦ Participation may lead to coercion by neighbours.
♦ Participation may raise expectations that cannot be fulfilled.
♦ Participation may lead to conflict.
♦ Participation may lead to development of agendas which do not match national or international development goals (McKee, 1993).

Long (1995), in a review of community participation in relationship to community based health programmes, stated that one of the most difficult tasks in community programmes is the mobiliza-

tion of community participation. Community members can often perceive that participation in programmes costs too much. Also, people begin to ask the question 'why do you want us to work so hard without pay?' Voluntarism is a major issue in community development programmes. In some societies, it is regarded as an appropriate and positive contribution and carries with it enhanced social roles. In other societies, voluntarism is regarded as a negative experience, in which the community regards unpaid work as inappropriate and demeaning. An understanding of community values is critical in determining the extent to which strategies for voluntarism will be cost-effective.

Participation in community development is also influenced to a great extent by the degree to which the community members identify with the topic or objective of the programme. In some community health activities, communities have stated that the care of disabled and disadvantaged individuals is primarily the responsibility of the extended family, and that community responsibility is only secondary.

It is also possible that the lack of knowledge regarding health and disability issues can create a situation where the community regards disability and health issues as 'dangerous'. An example of this would be the misconception that a disability may be transferable to others. Also, participation in programmes related to health and disability can create the problem of the volunteer not being respected as they have become associated with a minority or disadvantaged group. The development of community based rehabilitation in leprosy is an example of a programme in which the stigma and fear of the disease has a major impact on community participation.

Those who are protected by position and socioeconomic status sometimes fail to recognize the risks that community members take by participating in community disability programmes. Long (1995) stated that 'a truly participatory community programme that focuses upon the poorer and more vulnerable members of a community will eventually confront those who have a stake in maintaining the status quo'. Identification with marginal groups carries a risk.

Many organizers of community programmes are sensitive to the problems and difficulties associated with participation. As one particular approach to participation may not, on its own, be successful, a combination of strategies might be considered.

Kaleidoscopic Strategies

Each community is a kaleidoscope in itself, ever changing in its pattern. The patterns are determined by the way it is 'turned' when one looks at it and with each turn, the pieces fall into a new pattern. This is true also of the organization and nature of community development. Rather than continue to search for a single pattern that would capture the complexity of community dynamics, it may be appropriate to consider different patterns for different purposes (Long, 1995).

This kind of strategy can include building a community based programme on to an existing successful activity. An example of this is the successful addition of strategies for identifying disability in children to the activities of a maternal and child health, baby weighing station (Rohde, 1995). Participation can also be facilitated by encouraging coalitions of community and special interest groups. The collaboration between groups representing the physically disabled and visually and hearing impaired groups in Jamaica, which resulted in the Combined Disabilities Association, created a more effective national coalition for all its members.

Community participation is crucial to any effective community programme. To succeed, the activities must share the priorities of the target communities, utilize established community leaders as promoters and involve community members in the design, implementation and evaluation of activities.

REFERENCES

Borkensha, D. and Hodge, P. (1969) Community development: An interpretation. In *Social and Economic Change*. Chandler Publishing Company, San Francisco, California.

Bulmer, M., Lewis, J. and Piachaud, D. (1989) Social policy: the community-based approach. In *The Goals of Social Policy*. Unwin Hyman, London.

Helander, E. (1993) *Prejudice and Dignity, An Introduction to Community Based Rehabilitation. United Nations Development Program*, New York.

International Labour Organization (ILO), United Nations Educational, Scientific and Cultural Organization (UNESCO), World Health Organization (WHO) (1994) *Joint Position Paper on Community Based Rehabilitation for and with People with Disabilities*. Geneva: WHO.

Long, W. M. (1995) Community participation: where the ideal is unattainable we turn to the possible. Community participation in practice. *News on Health Care in Developing Countries* 4/95, **9**: 4–7.

McKee, N. (1993) Lessons for communicators. In *Social Mobilization and Social Marketing*. Southbound Penang, Malaysia.

Oxford English Dictionary (1975) Oxford University Press, Ely House, London.

Poplin, D. E. (1972) *Communities: A Survey of Theories and Methods Research*. Macmillan Company, New York.

Rifkin, S. B., Muller, F. and Bichman W. (1988) *Primary health care: on measuring community participation. Social Science and Medicine*. **26**: 931–940.

Rohde, J. (1995) Indonesia's Posyandus: Accomplishments and future challenges.

Community participation in practice. *News on Health Care in Developing Countries* 4/95, **9**: 40–47.

Stone, L. (1990) Cultural influence in community participation in health. *Social Science and Medicine* **35**(4): 409–417.

United Nations Development Program (UNDP) (1991) Division of Global and Interregional Programs. *Disabled People's Participation in Sustainable Human Development.*

Woelk, G.B. (1992) Cultural and structural influences in the creation of participation in community health programs. *Social Science and Medicine* **35**(4): 419–424.

World Health Organization Technical Report (1991) *WHO Study Report on Community Involvement in Health.* WHO, Geneva.

chapter four

Community Based Rehabilitation

INTRODUCTION TO COMMUNITY BASED REHABILITATION

Over the last twenty years community based rehabilitation (CBR) has emerged in economically disadvantaged countries as an effective method of providing rehabilitation services to more of the population, where the existing health and social services were unable to meet the demands of the disabled community and their families. The concept was based on a community development model and empowered persons with disabilities and their communities. The core characteristics of the different approaches to CBR have been shaped by a variety of social, economic and cultural conditions affecting the development, implementation and sustainability of health and social programmes.

Within the last decade, many economically advanced or developed countries have become increasingly aware of their own limitations in providing the broad spectrum of health and social services necessary to advance the rights of disabled persons. The increasing costs of institutional services in all aspects of health care have motivated governments and agencies to develop community programmes as a viable alternative to conventional institutional services. In addition, as political awareness of persons with disabilities has increased, CBR has evolved as an attractive and feasible strategy. There is an increasing recognition that traditional hospital and physician driven systems are not necessarily the most appropriate, socially acceptable or cost-effective approaches to service delivery. The changes brought about as part of the development of CBR emphasized the role of the family and community in the rehabilitation process. Another aspect of CBR is its focus on the integration of disabled persons in all aspects of community life, thereby enhancing the participation of disabled people in their communities. The development of CBR has also been influenced by the social movement toward the protection and promotion of human rights (Helander, 1995b).

Historically the attitudes, beliefs and behaviours of non-disabled persons have determined the opportunities and quality of life available to the community of dis-

Five Reactions to Persons with Disabilities.

- *Elimination* – removing the disabled from the community.
- *The 'poor house' approach* – removing them from view.
- *Institutional care* – segregation.
- *Integration* – the process leading to the full involvement of disabled persons in the life of their families, communities and society.
- *Self-actualization* – the ability of the disabled person to fulfil his or her need for living a life in dignified independence with self-esteem.

Figure 4.1

Institutional Based Rehabilitation Approaches.
Institutional rehabilitation – main features (adapted from Helander, 1993).

- Designed and controlled by professional groups
- Delivered by professionals
- Centralized
- Referral based
- Specialized
- Resources and technology intensive

Figure 4.2

abled persons. Helander (1993) stated that an 'alternative reaction to the presence of human beings with disabilities can be grouped under five main headings' (Figure 4.1).

HISTORICAL REVIEW

Institutional Services

The development and delivery of health and social services in the twentieth century were based on the 'medical model' of health care. This approach reinforced the role of the physician as the primary decision-maker and the individual who was regarded as having the knowledge to speak on behalf of persons with disability and their families (Figure 4.2). There was limited consultation between health care providers and their clients up to, and following, the period of the Second World War.

The scientific developments in rehabilitation medicine and related disciplines focused primarily on the development of institutional practice and services. This was also seen in the allocation of resources for the establishment and maintenance of specialist hospitals and centres specifically dealing with acute and chronic disability cases. The research environment also focused on the technological advancement of rehabilitation practice.

Institutional practice reinforced the development of special institutions dealing with unique populations of persons with disabilities, such as people with visual and hearing impairments, or those with chronic disabilities who would remain in institutions throughout their lives. In addition, people with certain disabilities, such as leprosy, mental handicaps and tuberculosis, were stigmatized and segregated.

Institutional practice in rehabilitation fell under scrutiny during the 1960s by organizations of rehabilitation professionals and international agencies including the World Health Organization. Concerns were related to the absence or gross inadequacy of rehabilitation services in developing countries and the over-concentration of resources in the institutional health care sector in developing societies (WHO, 1976). In addition, the lack of adequate services was now being reviewed in the context of the rapidly expanding population in need.

The lack of general accessibility to services was related to the concentration of resources in urban centres and the inability of economically disadvantaged countries to provide even basic rehabilitation services to all citizens. It also became apparent that the increasing competition for financial resources was further limiting the development of services for the disabled person and their communities. For the most part, the development of international health and social policies ignored the needs of persons with disabilities up to the time of the declaration by the United Nations of the Decade of the Disabled (1983 to 1992). This declaration has had a major influence on the general public and governments on issues related to the needs of disabled persons.

In the early 1970s, WHO reviewed its disability and rehabilitation policies. In 1976 the World Health Assembly adopted a resolution on disability prevention and rehabilitation which made a strong case for increasing resource allocations for disability programmes (WHO, 1977). Subsequent to these declarations there was an increase in the development of international programmes related to disability prevention and management. In the mid 1970s, WHO provided evidence to show that in disadvantaged societies a relatively large proportion of the health problems known to cause disability were preventable. Factors which influenced the disability rate included the lack of immunization, malnutrition and accidents.

Original Impetus for Community Based Rehabilitation

The international strategy of community based rehabilitation began in less developed regions of the world as early as the 1950s mainly because the idea made sense. The medical rehabilitation approach was too expensive and only met the needs of relatively few for a limited period of time. In the 1970s WHO and UNICEF promoted the idea of community health workers. The concept of community workers came about from a focus on poverty, health, development, population growth, and community involvement. In response to WHO's lead, many less developed countries initiated volunteer schemes and provided financial support by increasing rural health budgets.

One of the most significant policy developments by WHO in the 1970s was the development and implementation of CBR (WHO, 1976). The CBR concept was based on the concept that family members were the best resource in dealing with the daily needs of disabled persons as much of rehabilitation strategy is common sense and repetitive in nature. In order to enhance understanding of the concepts and practices related to CBR, a study of developing countries was undertaken by the WHO (Helander *et al.*, 1989). This study confirmed that persons with a disability were economically and socially disadvantaged in society and a large proportion of those who were born disabled did not survive beyond childhood.

At the same time, there were illustrations of spontaneous indigenous rehabilitation where communities and families started to rehabilitate their own family members. The development of CBR was accelerated by the work of Helander and colleagues (1989) with the distribution of a manual entitled *Training in the Community for People with Disabilities*. Designed for persons with disability, their families and community members, this manual was a major factor in the advancement, development and application of indigenous technology and the use of community personnel. Resource material was divided into a number of training packages, with guides to make it easier to understand and apply.

CBR training manuals such as *Training in the Community for People with Disabilities* (Helander *et al.*, 1989) have been used in more than thirty countries throughout the world and have been translated into a number of languages and dialects. The handbooks map out the process of transferring simplified rehabilitation techniques to persons with disabilities themselves, their families or caregivers, and community members. The process includes training individuals in the community in a workshop format to become 'local supervisors', who then perform a vital community service by communicating their expertise to members of the local community, with the objective of developing a network of primary care rehabilitation workers (McColl and Paterson, 1995).

DEFINING THE CONCEPT OF COMMUNITY BASED REHABILITATION

In the evolution of CBR a number of attempts have been made to define CBR in a way that encompasses its core elements or characteristics. The following is a selection of some of these definitions:

♦ *Community based rehabilitation is a strategy within community development for the rehabilitation, equalization of opportunities and social integration of all people with disabilities. CBR is implemented through the combined efforts of disabled people themselves, their families and communities and the appropriate health, education, vocational and social services* (ILO, UNESCO, WHO, 1994).
♦ *Community based rehabilitation is a strategy for enhancing the quality of life of disabled people by improving service delivery, by providing more*

equitable opportunities and by promoting and protecting their human rights (Helander, 1995a).
♦ *Community based rehabilitation is a comprehensive and holistic approach in the field of rehabilitation building on local resources, and enabling social integration of people with disabilities into the mainstream. The long-term significance of CBR is based on social change and total community development, rather than on mere services* (NORAD Seva-in-Action, 1992).
♦ Miles (1995) stated that the term community based rehabilitation is currently used in at least six distinguishable ways with some overlap.
  – *CBR is therapy or special measures given by families to disabled members in their homes with efforts to influence public attitudes and improve access to services. These efforts may be supported by a volunteer or paid worker.*
  – *CBR is therapeutic, educational, vocational or social self-help projects organized by disabled persons and their partners – with or without external technical help.*
  – *CBR is an ideology whereby a nation's entire resources for rehabilitation are centrally planned and allocated equitably across the population.*
  – *CBR is the provision of community programmes by rehabilitation institutions where resource centres take knowledge and skills to isolated or deprived communities (outreach).*
  – *CBR is an externally supported system in which trained and paid (CBR field workers) undertake the mobilization, training and public education tasks related to disability*
  – *CBR is the adoption of the term CBR by those not actively involved in community development and by organizations or institutions*

wishing to appear to conform to the latest 'trend' while actually continuing previous programme strategies.

Miles also states that an alternative approach called 'information based rehabilitation' focuses on how information – broadly understood as concepts, knowledge, skills, design and feedback – is created, transmitted, developed, monitored, applied, circulated and evaluated in these strategies (Miles, 1994).

THE CHANGING IDEOLOGY OF COMMUNITY BASED REHABILITATION – A SPIRIT OF TOLERANCE

In the early development of CBR the concept was owned to some degree by grassroots organizations, most frequently in the non-government sector and in economically disadvantaged societies. The initiatives were carried out by community members and persons with disabilities with little or no support or interest from the health professions. The last decade has shown, however, that much can be learned, and has been learned and applied from the early development of CBR and the basic principles underlying its evolution – community participation and sharing.

It has also been recognized that different cultures and different societies, including the economically advanced nations, will take from the concepts of CBR those strategies and approaches most appropriate for them. An international review of CBR shows that it now encompasses a range of services and programmes and it is part of a continuum of shared responsibility with other health and social agencies. CBR is no longer an adversary of the rehabilitation institution or agency. It is part of a broader relationship extending from the community to the specialist health care rehabilitation facility. This more global approach supports the concept of the sharing and maximizing of resources. CBR and its success has been a major influence in drawing the institution and its human resource base toward the community and in sensitizing the previously isolated medical model practitioners that they are also part of the continuum.

COMPOSITION OF COMMUNITY BASED REHABILITATION

General Principles of CBR

The term community based rehabilitation is now in use internationally with several different meanings. As societies differ in culture, environment, education, health and social programmes, so do their definitions of, and approaches to, CBR differ. There is no single approach that can be set apart as 'absolute CBR'. However, there is some consensus around the general principles of CBR (Peat and Boyce, 1993) (Figure 4.3).

Common Elements of Community Based Rehabilitation Programmes

As previously stated, at this time there is no single conclusive definition of CBR. However, some consensus has been reached on its general principles and components:

CBR programmes attempt to:

• change community attitudes and behaviours towards disability;
• empower persons with disabilities, enabling them to function in the community;

> **General Principles of Community Based Rehabilitation.**
> - Community and client centred
> - Focused on prevention and early intervention
> - Collaborators with institutional facilities
> - Promoters of consumer participation and control
> - Consistent and flexible
> - Coordinated by a referral system (lay referral systems are encouraged)
> - Interdisciplinary, multisectoral
> - Focused on information sharing
> - Agents to increase knowledge of contact people
> - Providers of appropriate knowledge to the community
> - Agents for selecting appropriate technology to fit community need
> - Providers of full- or part-time professional or non-professional teams appropriate to need

Figure 4.3

- transfer appropriate rehabilitation knowledge and skills to the community;
- assist in the change from users of services to participants in health programmes;
- establish partnership in the development and implementation of programmes
- translate appropriate clinical knowledge to self-help skills
- increase level of knowledge of contact people
- develop appropriate rehabilitation services.

Stakeholders in Community Based Rehabilitation

There are eight main stakeholders in any CBR programme:

- persons with disabilities;
- the family or caregivers of persons with disabilities;
- the community;
- volunteers;
- community health workers;
- rehabilitation professionals;
- multilateral and non-government organizations;
- employers.

Persons with Disabilities

A goal of CBR is to rehabilitate, educate and empower persons with disabilities, enabling them to integrate into their communities as productive, contributing members. In the CBR model, persons with disabilities themselves are active partners in the rehabilitation effort.

Family or Caregivers

In CBR, family members or caregivers are trained in providing simple rehabilitation services to persons with disabilities, and are encouraged to be creative about the use of simple aids and devices enabling persons with disabilities to function as contributing family members. Up to 90% of all personal assistance to the elderly and persons with disability comes from family members and caregivers and not from formal programmes. Women are the major caregivers in all societies and frequently have to balance this role with other family responsibilities and work outside the home. Although many women and families support the concept of elderly and disabled persons remaining in the home and community, they often feel inadequately supported (Gloag, 1985). Disabled individuals in a variety of cultures express their preference to live at home. However, many children with disabilities will outlive their family caregivers and require community support services in order for them to be maintained in the community (Peat and Boyce, 1993).

Community

CBR promotes the concept of community responsibility for health. Rehabilitation services are provided or managed by specially trained volunteers and workers from within the community. Communities are encouraged to 'take ownership' of CBR programmes.

Volunteers

Volunteer work in helping the poor, sick, disabled and needy is a known tradition in all cultures and societies throughout history. Frequently, volunteers in communities tend to be women. Volunteering can be defined as any act that is offered by persons without pay. The duties and contributions of volunteers in community based rehabilitation projects vary according to the complex economic, socio-cultural and motivational factors in any CBR environment. It has been suggested that programmes with a large number of community volunteers are those with the greatest potential for community control and ownership (Lysack, 1992).

Programmes that rely significantly on volunteers are vulnerable to the fluctuating motivation and interest of the participants. In some instances when financial payment is being made to other programme personnel, volunteers have questioned whether they should participate without financial compensation. The personal participation of volunteers or the 'in-kind' contribution of the individual cannot be separated from the impact that volunteering has on the community as a whole, and subsequently the use and allocation of community resources.

Community Workers

Community based rehabilitation seeks to improve the health of communities in general using a community development approach, which assumes that many of the needs of most persons with disabilities can be met through programmes that use appropriately trained non-professional personnel as well as professionals. Non-professional workers may be any member of the community, including handicapped and disabled people and their families. It has been observed that community workers who have disabilities themselves provide role models for other persons with disabilities in the community, giving hope and new vision to families and communities for the future. People with disabilities are likely to be more dedicated, committed to, and understanding of the solutions to problems as well as the societal obstacles and the struggle associated with disablement. However, persons with disabilities who assume community worker roles need to be cautioned so that they do not inadvertently function in such a way as to give one person authority over another (Helander, 1993).

Rehabilitation Professional Personnel

Rehabilitation professionals are an important resource in the development of CBR and can act as 'agents of change', by transferring basic skills and knowledge in the management of disability, and coordinating group efforts. To be effective, they must be specially educated with regard to their role in community programmes.

Governments and Multilateral Agencies

A major role of the health and social agencies at both the government and multilateral level is to provide public awareness and health promotion programmes which will enhance the understanding of disability issues and disability prevention in the general population (Peat and Boyce, 1993).

Employers

In terms of disability identification and management, it is important to link CBR to vocational rehabilitation initiatives which lead to the reintegration of persons with a disability into their communities and to their complete participation in the social and economic activities of daily life.

STRENGTHS AND WEAKNESSES OF COMMUNITY BASED REHABILITATION

Many individuals and agencies believe that CBR is the preferred approach to disability prevention, detection and intervention. There are, however, some distinct advantages and disadvantages to the approach. The following is a summary of some of these advantages and disadvantages based in part on the report of the NORAD Workshop *Sharing Strengths Seva-in-Action* (1992).

Advantages of Community Based Rehabilitation

- Wide service coverage that can be achieved.
- Community interaction and empowerment.
- Affordability/cost-effectiveness.
- Build-up of manpower resources.
- Comprehensive and holistic development.
- Promotion of awareness/acceptance.
- Sustainability.
- Wise use of local resources.
- Needs-based planning.
- Partnership involving stakeholders in programme development and implementation (*ICACBR Update*, 1993).

Disadvantages of Community Based Rehabilitation

- The dilution of care which can result from a lack of specialized training for service providers.
- Difficulties with evaluation.
- Possibility of reducing the importance of professional services.
- Problems in realizing decentralization.
- Unreliability of community involvement.
- Potential for government denial of responsibility for service provision.
- Limitations of local resources.
- Difficulties in large-scale cooperation/ coordination (*ICACBR Update*, 1993).

A DESCRIPTIVE FRAMEWORK OF COMMUNITY BASED REHABILITATION

McColl and Paterson (1995) have taken the continuum approach further so that it can be used as a tool for learning from the diversity of CBR programmes. Along an individual/community continuum, McColl and Paterson use consistent factors to capture features that define and support CBR programmes.

Factors that Define CBR Programmes
- Aims
- Beneficiaries
- Strategies

These are either individually focused (on the person with the disability and his or her family), or community focused (those directed to the community as a whole).

Aims
The aims of a CBR programme include what the programme intends to achieve and what observable changes it actually brings about.
Individually focused aims include:

- direct service – to people with disabilities and their families;
- family support – to caregivers;

♦ vocational development;
♦ empowerment – greater awareness of issues related to disability.

Community focused aims include:

♦ attitude change – to sensitize the community toward the special needs of persons with disabilities;
♦ sustainability – to develop a sustainable network of CBR resources and to integrate these with existing health, social, vocational and developmental programmes;
♦ advocacy – to organize people with disabilities and encourage them to become pressure groups to influence policy;
♦ education of existing and future professionals – to encourage an understanding of CBR strategies and to incorporate CBR into the curriculum of rehabilitation professionals;
♦ research – analysis of the theoretical, academic and practical knowledge base.

Beneficiaries
The second defining dimension describes 'the people and organizations that benefit from the existence of the programme'. Beneficiaries, like aims, are described along a continuum from individuals to community.
    Individual beneficiaries include:

♦ individuals with disabilities;
♦ families of individuals with disabilities;

Community beneficiaries include:

♦ the community as a whole;
♦ multisectoral programmes that work with a variety of professionals (teachers, religious leaders, government officials, organizations, and agencies).

Strategies
A third defining dimension describes the strategies 'that CBR programmes use to achieve their aims'. Strategies may be individually or community focused.
    Individually oriented strategies include:

♦ providing information – such as training families in simplified rehabilitation techniques;
♦ developing organization – clinicians, person with disability and family work together to define and meet goals;
♦ accessing resources – finding support groups for people with disabilities and their families;
♦ providing technological aids – for people with disabilities and their families.

Community   oriented   strategies include:

♦ providing information – such as a field worker training community members by telling them about the referral system; by giving communities information on making communities accessible in terms of pavements, banks, recreational facilities, etc.;
♦ developing organization – by encouraging the community team to develop their own systems; by helping the community find out what people with disabilities need so that the community can continue the programme;
♦ accessing resources – by involving local volunteer professionals, political leaders, non-government organizations (NGOs); by communities generating their own funds;
♦ developing leadership – by creating positive role models of people with disabilities.

Factors that Support CBR Programmes
♦ Human resources
♦ Structural resources
♦ Attitudes

Human resources

Human resources are potentially the most important resource for any community development programme. These can be from within the community itself, or obtained from an external source.

Within the community:

♦ 'people with or without prior association with the service sector, whose expertise is marshalled for the benefit of disabled community members';
♦ consumers, people with disabilities (farmers, teachers, religious leaders, volunteers).

Outside the community include:

♦ health professionals (including physicians, physiotherapists and occupational therapists);
♦ strategic planners and lobbyists.

Structural resources

Structural resources are the organizations, institutions, and groups that offer tangible resources (other than personnel) which act as important sustainers of the programmes because of the role they play in continued operation.

Inside the community include:

♦ existing community groups or institutions – use the existing infrastructure;
♦ municipal or local government – strengthen liaisons; use existing facilities;
♦ local service clubs, business, or industries – employ people with disabilities.

Outside the community include:

♦ government connections;
♦ educational programmes;
♦ health services and institutions;
♦ NGOs and community groups.

Attitudes

The third supporting factor is attitudes 'that have the potential to have an impact on the shape and structure and success of a programme'. Attitudes may originate within the community or outside it, and may be friendly or hostile toward people with disabilities.

Attitudes within the community:

♦ positive image – a person with a disability is economically self-sufficient, living with dignity, contributing to community development;
♦ negative image – pity, sympathy and not much faith in what people with disabilities can achieve.

Attitudes outside the community:

♦ positive attitudes – are often linked to the availability of more and better information about disability;
♦ negative attitudes – often reflect widely held social and cultural stereotypes about disability, such as social stigmas, hidden sense of shame regarding disability.

THE CONTINUUM

Rehabilitation extends from the individual in the community to the institution, and should be viewed as a dynamic continuum. While the two concepts of institutional based rehabilitation and community based rehabilitation are often presented as mutually exclusive, they are actually two components of a single continuum. Figure 4.4 shows that the two can operate interdependently – that CBR is not a categorical concept, and is best characterized by the overall degree and distribution of rehabilitation strategies.

← ——————————————— **THE CONTINUUM** ——————————————— →

Acute care and specialist facility	Outreach services	Home care programme	Social services	Community workers	Volunteers	Family/ caregiver	Person with disability

INSTITUTIONAL
BASED
REHABILITATION

COMMUNITY
BASED
REHABILITATION

Figure 4.4 The continuum.

COMMUNITY BASED REHABILITATION STRATEGY

CBR provides the basic level rehabilitation strategies to be delivered to individuals and their families in a way that does not rely heavily on professionals, institutions, external resources and technology. CBR programmes use local resources as building blocks to form networks of lay people trained in aspects of rehabilitative care. Community members increase their knowledge, skill and understanding of disability issues. Vocational skill development and income generating activities for persons with disabilities are often included in CBR programmes (Peat and Boyce, 1993). Perhaps what is most important is that CBR enhances social awareness and interest. In the CBR process persons with disabilities are more likely to maximize their physical and mental abilities, and have opportunities to achieve full social integration within their communities. In turn, communities have a new potential to view people with disabilities as competent contributors to community life.

The common denominator of CBR activities is that each approach is different. The difference is to be expected, because CBR should reflect the communities where it exists, and communities themselves are always different from one another (Pupulin, 1995). As Pupulin stated:

Where CBR projects are in conflict, it is not because of differences in communities, but because of differences in the ideology of the people who initiated the project, and who have not allowed the communities to have control of the activities.

'Bottom-up' or 'Top-down' Approaches to CBR

The supporters of the 'bottom-up' approach to CBR believe that 'grassroots' community rehabilitation is not only the most appropriate, it is the original and exclusive approach to CBR. Contrary to its own ideology, this approach can involve an outside stimulus and often functions well if there is a charismatic leader at the community level (Pupulin, 1995). Unfortunately, in some instances, these projects are not sustainable because the community cannot maintain CBR without the collaboration and support of established health and social agencies.

The 'top-down' approach to CBR implies the involvement of health and social agencies or individuals outside the community in the design and provision of community programmes. Many societies have debated the issue of 'community action' versus 'government control' in their health and social services. However, it is now recognized that there is a need for partnership between communities and established health and social agencies in order to ensure that communities have the responsibility for their members, and that the health and social agencies provide the relevant support (Oakley, 1989). What may be most desirable is an approach which combines aspects of both the 'bottom-up' and 'top-down' approaches, an approach that is both appropriate and sustainable.

THE COMMUNITY ORIENTED APPROACH TO REHABILITATION

Community based rehabilitation and community oriented, institutional based rehabilitation (IBR) are both part of a continuum extending from the person with disability and the family through to the specialized service institution. CBR and IBR are not mutually exclusive and both can be considered part of one rehabilitation system, interacting in a multisectoral fashion to provide services at various levels, appropriate to the nature of disability and the organization of health and social programmes.

Eldar (1994) stated that in order to assume responsibility for rehabilitation at the community level, primary health care (PHC) should be supported by rehabilitation institutions, and reoriented to assist in the assessment of disability, the provision of initial treatment and the training and education of primary care teams in the management of disabled persons. A rehabilitation institution that practises 'community oriented rehabilitation' (COR) would be optimally able to perform this role.

The community served by COR is an aggregation of disabled and elderly whose care would normally be the responsibility of primary care providers. The term can be applied to a geographically defined population or confined to members of a health insurance plan, or a health maintenance organization. COR services might be located in an institution that is located within the boundaries of the community, for instance the rehabilitation department of a local community hospital, general hospital, regional rehabilitation facility or a national referral centre. All activities of an institution practising COR are conducted in full cooperation with the PHC system, consisting of family physicians, clinical specialists, community nurses, and other health professionals and social workers at the community level (Eldar, 1994).

The institution involved in COR would:

♦ provide comprehensive inpatient day care and/or outpatient rehabilitation services;
♦ exhibit a concern with mental and social, as well as physical, health;
♦ have a willingness to reach into the community to identify those in need
♦ have a readiness to develop new services at the institutional and community level;
♦ involve the community in the care of the disabled and elderly and in the formation of voluntary organizations and self-help groups;
♦ educate primary care teams and the disabled and elderly and their caregivers in rehabilitation.

Programmes that lend themselves to the community oriented approach include:

♦ clinical rehabilitation;
♦ outreach activities;
♦ patient and family education;
♦ community participation;

♦ education and training;
♦ interagency cooperation;
♦ environmental modifications.

The above describes a system in which COR is implemented as an integrated system of rehabilitation in which the rehabilitation facility, primary and secondary care services and other resources at the community level collaborate to increase the availability and accessibility of rehabilitation services. Successful COR is the integration of a rehabilitation institution with primary care and elements of secondary care into one system, focusing on disability issues.

SERVICE STRATEGIES FOR COMMUNITY BASED REHABILITATION

In a number of countries rehabilitation services are currently available within the framework of existing services.

Community outreach from hospital
In this approach, community services are made available either through a 'satellite' community clinic or directly, by hospital based personnel providing a community service. Institutional based outreach programmes include travelling clinics for paediatric rehabilitation, regional brain injury outpatient services and mobile clinics established by a rehabilitation centre to provide follow-up services in the home environment The satellite clinic model is used by the 'sveti Duh' hospital, in Zagreb, Croatia, where community rehabilitation services are made available at a separately located facility in a densely populated urban area. The staff provide clinic and outreach services focusing on a variety of clinical areas including traumatic head injury, musculoskeletal trauma and rehabilitation of war victims. Another example is in Bombay, where clinical staff from King Edward Memorial Hospital provide direct community services in an urban community located in a heavily industrialized area. The clinical staff do not operate a satellite clinic, but provide direct home visiting outreach services.

Outreach programmes draw on the specialized rehabilitation resources of urban centres and the delivery of these resources or services to under-serviced communities. In contrast, CBR programmes focus on developing rehabilitation resources at the community level. In other words, while outreach programmes and community oriented programmes are 'for' the community, they are not 'of ' the community. Outreach is a strategy that has been developed by specialized rehabilitation services developing community programmes in disadvantaged or under-serviced areas. In many instances, outreach programmes focus on the needs of rural communities. However, they can also be used to provide services to disadvantaged communities in urban centres. While meeting the immediate needs of the community, these programmes do not solve the problem of how to integrate the community into the design and delivery of the programmes (Peat and Boyce, 1993).

Outreach programmes can be either 'institutionally based' or 'network system' programmes. The primary distinguishing characteristic between these types of programmes is whether or not they are based in urban rehabilitation institutions.

Network outreach
This service provides interdisciplinary professional support directly in the home. In many parts of the province of Ontario in Canada these services have no institutional base, and may operate entirely from a central planning or admin-

istration base whose sole function is programme management. The Home Care programme in Kingston, Canada operates on this basis and provides occupational therapy, physical therapy and nursing services for a wide variety of clinical needs including early discharge from hospital, long-term chronic illness, and geriatric care. Another example is the Arthritis Society of Canada, who provide home visiting programmes dealing with a specific disability issue.

Community rehabilitation clinic
The reduction in institutional services caused by the economic recession and restructuring of health and social programmes is moving a number of rehabilitation services out of the traditional hospital or institutional setting. Outpatient services which were once offered as part of a tertiary care institution are now being relocated to a community environment. The development of community rehabilitation facilities which provide outpatient services and focus primarily on ambulatory programmes is one of the aspects of the restructuring of the health care system in Alberta, Canada. These programmes provide multidisciplinary facilities located in the community and require no medical referral.

Rehabilitation services within primary health community centres
Primary health community centres which have traditionally offered a broad range of ambulatory clinical services, such as maternal and child health, have not traditionally included rehabilitation services. In the restructuring of health and social programmes in former Yugoslavia, rehabilitation is being provided in the existing 'Dom Zdravlji' (house of health) system. These primary health community centres include rehabilitation services to meet the needs of the community where the institutional base

is unable to meet the demand. The PHC system can be a very effective vehicle for providing services at a community level. These services can also be linked to 'home visiting' or 'outreach programmes' and to specialized services in the hospital sector.

Community vocational rehabilitation services
The International Labour Organization (ILO) has supported the development of a number of community vocational training programmes which focus on the vocational training and reintegration of persons with disabilities into the workforce.

Community programmes without professional health care associations
The history of CBR has been based on the provision of community based rehabilitation programmes which evolved at the grassroots level to provide a wide range of programmes for the disabled person and their caregivers and family. These programmes may not be linked with an existing professional rehabilitation service. The Disabled Farmers of Alberta is an organization which was developed by disabled farmers and had the primary objective of providing support and training for disabled farmers so that they could remain productive and active members of the farming community. Programmes address the overall needs of the individual from networking and information on professional rehabilitation services to obtaining appropriate personal and social support, adaptive technology and financial assistance.

Another example of this type of activity is the Kailas Foundation in Ellora, India. This is a community development group, organized by rural women to provide a wide range of social services, including support to disabled persons and their families.

SERVICE COORDINATION

Rehabilitation services are offered by different programmes, serving different groups and run by different agencies. Those who need services can find this confusing and time consuming. In addition, service programmes often have different eligibility criteria and service standards. The multisectoral approach emphasizes the need to match services to the needs of consumers and requires significant intersectoral cooperation (Peat and Boyce, 1993). The current development of CBR illustrates the advantages of a multisectoral approach to the design and implementation of programmes for persons with disabilities. A multisectoral approach coordinates health and social services, education, employment and integration strategies and the development of an information system in a way that ensures that people with disabilities know about the resources available and how to obtain them.

COMMUNITY BASED VOCATIONAL REHABILITATION AND THE INTERNATIONAL LABOUR ORGANIZATION (ILO)

Vocational rehabilitation services have been developed in a number of countries to assist a person with an injury or disability to return to work or prepare for new work and other activities. Vocational rehabilitation does not only focus on work. It also deals with the needs and requirements of the individual to return to a productive life. If an individual is unable to return to a paid job, vocational rehabilitation provides the opportunity to attend classes, learn new skills or be involved in voluntary activities. Vocational rehabilitation services are offered in many different settings depending on the community. Many are offered in hospitals, workplaces, schools and other community facilities.

Depending on personal circumstances, an individual with a disability may require assistance with the following:

♦ assessment of an individual's strengths and limitations, and their corresponding effect on the ability to work and manage in the home environment;
♦ coping with the injury or disability;
♦ education and training aimed at returning the individual to the workforce;
♦ recommendations on the physical changes that may be required to permit the individual to function in the workplace;
♦ recommendations on physical changes in the home to facilitate the activities of daily living.

Because vocational rehabilitation can involve many different levels of workers (manual labour to professional service) and several different services, it is often appropriate for the person with disabilities to involve a Coordinator of Services. This Coordinator would be someone who knows the details of the case and who will work to obtain the appropriate services. This person could be a physical therapist, occupational therapist, physician, rehabilitation counsellor, a person with a disability or an individual assigned by an insurance agency. A Coordinator can:

♦ review the assessment to develop a thorough understanding of the client's work skills and the areas for improvement;
♦ develop a job plan in partnership with the person with disability, based on knowledge of the current employment situation in the community;
♦ assist in locating resources and support available in the community;

- assist with locating income sources for the client during the period of vocational rehabilitation;
- assist with the development of a financial plan to meet the costs of the vocational rehabilitation services required through a combination of the following:
  - Workers Compensation Board;
  - group or individual disability insurance;
  - disability component of a pension plan;
  - governmental assistance;
  - the current personal resources of the client (ILO, 1996).

Momm and Konig (1989) state that most CBR programmes which have developed in recent years are inspired by the medical rehabilitation paradigm. The adult with a long-term disability who seeks vocational training and income generating opportunities requires a programme with an emphasis on training and employment. To apply the medical rehabilitation paradigm to training and employment services for disabled adults is misleading and may have implications which prevent, rather than advance, the reintegration of persons with disabilities into society. Health and rehabilitation agencies generally do not have the mandate nor the professional competence to deal effectively with vocational rehabilitation. Momm and Konig suggest that 'in order to prevent misunderstandings and confusion, it would therefore have been advisable to abandon the term CBR and instead, clearly distinguish between Community Based Medical Rehabilitation (CBMR) and Community Based Vocational Rehabilitation (CBVR)'.

The focus on rehabilitation has to be complemented by a focus on the equalization of opportunities for persons with disabilities, or activities other than rehabilitation which will play a critical role in the integration process. The essential part of the integration effort depends on the attitude of the community and its institutions, and their endorsement of the concept that disabled people should not be marginalized or segregated, but rather should be offered equal opportunities. In this strategy, rehabilitation services must invest more effort in ensuring that disabled people also receive services from non-rehabilitation community resources. There is a shift from rehabilitation to an advocacy type of promotional programme for persons with a disability. In this approach, the term 'community integration programme' (CIP) could replace the term CBR. This would be appropriate where a rehabilitation agency is setting up programmes geared to the equalization of training and employment opportunities and to the social integration of persons with disabilities.

STRATEGIES FOR CHANGES TOWARD COMMUNITY BASED REHABILITATION

Broadening the Definition of Health

Rehabilitation cannot view physical or mental health in isolation from the individual. The impact of vocational status, support networks, spirituality, cultural context, functional levels and much more need consideration. Rehabilitation programmes must present, maintain and promote a broader view of health. Health education curricula need to be examined to reveal the view of health that is transmitted to new professionals. Recognition and respect among professionals in the health-related disciplines and between these professionals and users of the health system are essential in establishing a comprehensive view of health.

Shift from Curative to Preventive, and the Promotion of Health

In the mid 1970s, the health professions increasingly acknowledged the advantages of community resources (such as midwives, informal support and residential living) and the appropriateness of many health actions that people undertook themselves. This changing emphasis was accompanied in the industrialized world by the movement in favour of self-care and support networks, and increasing public awareness about lifestyle effects on health. This social movement facilitated the shift away from a reactive medical system of 'cure only' to one which promoted health and prevented disease. This shift is dependent on the acknowledgement of a broader definition of health and health maintenance.

Switching Focus from Specialized to Community Based Care

There is a Native North American saying that reflects the importance of participation: 'Tell me, and I'll forget. Show me and I may remember. Involve me, and I'll understand.' This 'understanding' is what may facilitate successful rehabilitation. The client-centred holistic philosophy of rehabilitation requires that the role of the consumer or person with disability be considered in all aspects of treatment. An ability to function adequately and enjoy a certain quality of life within the community must be established by the client. This switch from institutional rehabilitation to community rehabilitation does not, however, imply a severing of ties with professionals in urban institutions. Rather, community care providers will have to look to a centralized system (institutions) for support.

Providing More Opportunities for Consumers to Participate with Service Providers in Making Decisions on Health Choices and Policies

Historically, the participation of consumers in the health care system has not been encouraged. The political concept of empowerment is a component of the disability movement which has helped identify this neglect and promotes the involvement of consumers in programmes.

PROFESSIONAL AND BUREAUCRATIC CHALLENGES

While rehabilitation professionals have developed augmented roles with specialization in institutional sectors, community rehabilitation practice has been mostly ignored at the undergraduate and graduate levels of professional education. Thus, the ability of institutionally trained professionals to understand and meet the needs of a person with a disability living in the community may be limited. Unless professionals have had the opportunity to gain experience outside of the institutional setting, they may not develop the range of skills required to understand the needs of people in the context of the home and community environment.

While the rehabilitation professional possesses better knowledge regarding the expected effectiveness of rehabilitation therapy in improving health status, the individual knows best how improvements in health status will affect his or her well-being (Hurley et al., 1992). Policy-makers will take into consideration the knowledge base of both the professional and the individual in order to achieve an efficient allocation of rehabilitation resources.

Efficient allocation of resources will be achieved by:

♦ increasing the individual's/disabled person's knowledge of clinical effectiveness and the expected outcomes of therapeutic options;
♦ making the professional aware of, and sensitive to, the individual's preferences.

The role of the professional in the community is usually not to implement programmes, but to enhance the ability of persons with disabilities, their families and communities to achieve their own goals. It may be difficult for some professionals to let the 'professional as expert' role give way to the 'professional as consultant' role. Professional educational programmes should place a greater emphasis on teaching persons with disabilities and their families self-care instead of focusing solely on medical management. In general, there seems to be a growing awareness that the future development of CBR will depend to a large degree on the design, implementation and evaluation of educational strategies in the community environment.

The transfer of knowledge from professionals to non-professionals is one of the keys to the success of CBR. While this transfer has worked in many countries, generally the knowledge base in rehabilitation is considered to be the property of professionals and is not to be accessed or used by groups or individuals outside of the profession. Therefore, knowledge becomes private property and is owned, particularly in more developed countries where there is often formal protection marking territorial rights of individual professional disciplines. Territorial protection is often enforced through legislation governing scope of practice and is a legal and ethical barrier to the diffusion of knowledge to other professionals and non-professionals.

At the same time, it is known that community members provide an awareness of local needs and values, available resources, historical and political issues. Further, community volunteers may assume roles as fundraisers or advocates of policy. Participation of community members usually increases acceptability, visibility and accessibility of CBR initiatives and provides an essential base of knowledge promoting effective CBR.

The question of training and using community human resources is likely to remain a contentious issue in many countries. What many might view as loss of a professional mandate is likely to be viewed differently in different countries, as legislation governing education, training and employment varies. Many countries have taken substantial initiatives to work around the scope of practice issue by using the 'delegated acts' portion of the legislation to allow enhanced roles outside of the profession itself. One example of this is the introduction of the nurse practitioner and rehabilitation assistant in North America.

COMMUNITY BASED REHABILITATION IN AREAS OF CONFLICT AND PEACE BUILDING

Conflict in Bosnia-Herzegovina has resulted in a considerable number of people requiring rehabilitation services in the Sarajevo area. While some institutional rehabilitation programmes are functioning, a community based, low technology rehabilitation service is not generally available. Queen's University, Canada was requested by the government of Canada to collaborate with the World Health Organization (WHO) and other appropriate agencies in Sarajevo in the development of a programme proposal for a Canadian contribution to the enhancement of community based rehabilitation services.

The quality and scope of rehabilitation programmes available in Bosnia-Herzegovina has been seriously compromised by a shortage of health professionals who have experience in physical and occupational therapy. Not only have a significant number of professionals left the country, but those therapists that remain carry a caseload in excess of 50 outpatients a day, resulting in long hours of work.

The governments of Bosnia-Herzegovina want to develop community based rehabilitation within the primary health care system. This means that professional staff will be available at primary care centres to organize the treatment of individuals with disabilities. This is a shift in philosophy from the pre-war medical rehabilitation approach, when individuals with disabilities were 'treated' in large institutional centres. This shift is consistent with the international initiatives to provide adequate and appropriate services to individuals within a community framework. CBR has been particularly effective in meeting the demands of disabled communities and has been a strategy increasingly applied in the international restructuring of health and social programmes.

In the restructuring of health and social programmes in former Yugoslavia, rehabilitation is being provided in the existing 'Dom Zdravljas' (house of health) system. These primary health community centres include rehabilitation services to meet the needs of the community where the institutional base was unable to meet the demand. These 'houses of health' are actually health promoting institutions. The principles of health care ideology for Croatia listed in Figure 4.5 parallel WHO concepts, and reflect the inclusion of community participation in health care and the development of new roles for rehabilitation professionals.

The development and implementation of CBR in post-conflict periods is an effec-

Ten Principles of Health Care Ideology in Croatia (Stamper, 1995).

1. To keep the population informed is more important than to make laws.
2. It is most important to prepare a community to have a proper idea about health problems.
3. Questions concerning public health care and actions to be taken are not the physician's monopoly; everybody has to be engaged in solving them. Only joint efforts can improve public health.
4. A health care professional should be chiefly a social worker; individual treatment cannot achieve as much as when treatment is combined with social therapy.
5. A health care professional must not depend financially on his patients since it would prevent him from performing his duties.
6. When public health is in question, there must be no difference between the rich and the poor.
7. Health care should be organized so that the health care professional will seek out the patient not vice versa, because this is the only way to cover a large number of those for whose health we are responsible.
8. A health care professional should be teacher to the people.
9. Public health care is more important from an economic than from a humanitarian point of view.
10. A health care professional's first place is to be where people live. Secondary responsibilities are research and administration.

Figure 4.5

tive strategy in 'peace building' as it brings political, ethnic and social groups together to focus on a common goal – the rehabilitation of war victims and other disabled persons and their integration into a peaceful society. Rehabilitation as a peace-building strategy is seen in a wide variety of locations, including Bosnia-Herzegovina, Sri Lanka, Afghanistan, Cambodia and Angola.

In summary, the community based approach to rehabilitation emphasizes the use of simple technology, community involvement and teaching persons with disabilities and their families. This does not rule out the need for institutional care, but requires a continuum of services that are accessible and appropriate for the individual. Reintegration requires that services be provided in an equitable manner so that services are flexible and responsive to community needs.

REFERENCES

Eldar, R. (1994) *Community Oriented Rehabilitation (COR)*. Loewenstein Hospital Rehabilitation Centre, Raanana, Israel.

Gloag, D. (1985) Severe disability: Residential care and living in the community. *British Medical Journal* **290**: 368–371.

Helander, E. (1993) *Prejudice and Dignity: An Introduction to Community Based Rehabilitation*. United Nations Development Program, New York.

Helander, E. (1995a) CBR concept and principles – a historical perspective. *NU News on Health Care in Developing Countries* 2/95, **9**: 6–10.

Helander, E. (1995b) *Disabled People's Participation in Sustainable Human Development*. United Nations Development Program, Geneva.

Helander, E., Mendis, P., Nelson, G. and Goerdt, A. (1989) *Training in the Community for People with Disabilities*. WHO, Geneva.

ICACBR Update (1993) International Centre for the Advancement of Community Based Rehabilitation, Kingston, Canada **1**(2).

Hurley, J., Birch, S. and Eyles, J. (1992) *Information, Efficiency and Decentralization within Health Care Systems*. CHEPA Working Paper Series, No. 92–91. McMaster University, Hamilton, Ontario.

International Labour Organization (1996) ILO home page, *Mandate*. www.ilo.org/english/overview/mandate/htm.

International Labour Organization (ILO), UNESCO, and the World Health Organization (WHO) (1994) *Joint Position Paper on Community Based Rehabilitation for and with People with Disabilities*. Geneva.

Lysack, C. (1992) *Community Based Rehabilitation and Volunteerism: An Indonesian Experience with Motivation of Volunteer Workers*. MSc. thesis. Queen's University, Kingston, Canada.

Lysack, C. and Krefting L. (1993). Community based rehabilitation cadres: their motivation for volunteerism. *International Journal of Rehabilitation Research* **16**: 133–141.

Miles, M. (1994) Information Based Rehabilitation and Research. Preliminary Paper, CBR Symposium, Bangalore, December 1994 based on Miles paper in 1993, Service development by information not ideology. In H. Finkerflugel (Ed.) *The Handicapped Community. The Relation between Primary Health Care and Community Based Rehabilitation*. VU University Press, Amsterdam.

Miles, M. (1995) Personal and informal communication with the author, of unpublished material on definitions of community based rehabilitation.

McColl, M. A. and Paterson, J. (1995) Final Report: Critical Dimensions of Community-Based Rehabilitation. Development of a Descriptive Framework for CBR, September. ICACBR, Kingston, Canada.

Momm, W. and Konig, A. (1989) *From Community Based Rehabilitation to Community Integration Programmes*. International Labour Office, WHO, Geneva.

NORAD (1992) *Sharing Strengths.* Workshop on Community Based Rehabilitation, with Seva-in-Action, Bangalore, India.

Oakley, P. (1989) *Community Involvement in Health Development, An Examination of the Critical Issues.* WHO, Geneva.

Peat, M. (1991) Community based rehabilitation: development and structure, Part 1. *Clinical Rehabilitation* 3: 219–227.

Peat, M. (1991) Community based rehabilitation: development and structure, Part 2. *Clinical Rehabilitation* 5: 231–239.

Peat, M. (1995) *Community Based Rehabilitation in Developed Countries.* ICACBR publication, Queen's University, Kingston, Canada.

Peat, M. and Boyce, W. (1993) Canadian community rehabilitation services: challenges for the future. *Canadian Journal of Rehabiliation* 6(4): 281–289.

Pupulin, E. (1995) The concept of Community Based Rehabilitation: reflexions on current status and future perspectives. *NU News on Health Care in Developing Countries* 2/95, **9**: 4–5.

Stamper, W. (1996) *Ten Principles of Health Care Ideology in Croatia.* Public document on Health Care System, government, Zagreb.

United Nations (1985) *World Program of Action Concerning Disabled Persons.* New York.

Walt G. (1987) Community involvement: In Halstead S. B., Walsh J. A. (eds). *Why Things Work – Case Histories in Development.* Proceedings of a conference held at the Bellagio Conference Centre, Bellagio, Italy, October.

World Health Organization (1976) *A29/INF.DOC/1.* WHO, Geneva.

World Health Organization (1981) Expert Committee on Disability Prevention and Rehabilitation. *WHO Technical Report* **68B**: 7–37.

chapter
five

Community Based Rehabilitation Models

In community based rehabilitation (CBR), persons with disabilities go through the process of rehabilitation in their homes and communities. The community is actively involved in the design and implementation of programmes and in the social integration of the disabled person. There are many approaches to the implementation of community programmes. Models of CBR are as diverse as the communities themselves.

Within the last decade the increasing appreciation of CBR has led to the development of a number of approaches to the implementation of community activities focusing on the needs of persons with disabilities. This diversity of approaches reflects the infinite variety of cultures, communities and resources that contribute to CBR. For this reason, there can be no 'single path to enlightenment' for CBR. It is important to view the diversity as a natural phenomenon in the rehabilitation development process.

DEFINING AND CLASSIFYING CBR MODELS

We began CBR as an idea which people used in different ways. But most people agree with the main idea – that people with disabilities should have a better life. But people have different ideas about how this should be done.

(Miles, 1994)

Debates surrounding what CBR is, or is not, are similar to those related to decentralization. The issue becomes embedded in broader ideological perspectives and then become somewhat emotionally charged. CBR and the decentralization of health and social programmes is seen by some as the key to empowering individuals and communities, increasing public participation and restoring a balance in a system perceived to have been co-opted by experts. As one observer noted, 'Decentralization has come to symbolize a value rather than a characteristic of an organization seeking the achievement of specific values' (Hurley *et al.*, 1992). These factors have often grounded the debate of CBR more in rhetoric (in the negative sense) than in an analytical or empirical investigation.

In the early stages of development, the relationship between community based rehabilitation and institutionally based rehabilitation was a source of some tension in the international CBR community. Avid promoters of CBR claimed that the community based approach was incompatible with the acute care institutional approach to service delivery. On the other hand, excluding the option of seeking institutional care denies the needs of people with newly acquired disabilities or those with acute medical complications resulting from existing disabilities, as these groups require time limited, resource intensive care. In hospital, when an individual is first faced with a disability and the magnitude of medical and psychological issues, there is an inherent willingness on the part of professionals to shoulder responsibility when they perceive that clients/individuals are truly not able to assume decision-making authority (McColl and Paterson, 1995).

Some within the community see the acute care or specialist institution as a provider of inpatient programmes. Outpatient or ambulatory services are frequently viewed as the supporting mechanism for inpatient services. The concept of hospital staff 'reaching out' by visiting a disabled person in the community is not what most hospital staff would regard as consistent with the hospital's mission, policies, resources or clinical programmes.

The institutional/community issue aside, some CBR activists are critical of the service orientation of CBR, claiming that CBR is about social change and community development, not 'mere services' (NORAD Seva-in-Action, 1992).

MODELS OF CBR

Since CBR programmes come in all shapes, sizes and packages it is difficult to put them into a perfectly defined set of CBR models. Classifying CBR is extremely difficult as the models are as varied as the communities they serve. A common feature of CBR is that any model must be specifically tailored to meet the needs and context of the sponsoring community. As communities differ from one another, so too do CBR programmes. A number of authors have attempted to understand and classify these differences by describing models of CBR (McColl and Paterson, 1995).

♦ *Aims*: Murthy and Gopalan (1992) described models of CBR based on the aims of the programme. Medical, educational, economic (vocational), community development, and finally comprehensive including other aims, such as a combination of the previous four.

♦ *Structure*: Peat and Boyce (1993) described community rehabilitation services focusing on the structural aspects of the programmes. Community services were classified as institutional, network and outreach. Non-service agencies are those that facilitate CBR but may not themselves offer direct clinical services.

♦ *Human resources*: Periquet (1989) described CBR in terms of the human resource base. This included non-professional (community members, persons with disabilities) semi-professionals (community workers), specialists or professionals.

♦ *Origin*: Kisanji (1995) classified CBR according to the origin of the programme, whether is is a national or regional government programme, or a programme developed by a non-government organization (and multi-sectoral organizations) either nationally or internationally, and community or individual (grassroots, persons with disabilities).

Although the models described above focus on different aspects of CBR, many of the models and taxonomies have some features in common and some that are unique. Perhaps the most evident observation about the review of models on CBR is the lack of any consensus around definitions.

Figure 5.1 shows the four broad categories introduced earlier.

Additional descriptive information is provided under the headings of Organization, Objectives and Activities.

In the rest of this chapter, these classifications are applied to existing CBR programmes. The point of this exercise is to show that there are many different visions of CBR, although all share the desire to shift the locus of rehabilitation strategies to local communities and/or to individuals with disabilities living in their communities.

Aims (Murthy and Gopalan, 1992)	Structure (Peat and Boyce, 1993)	Human resources (Periquet, 1989)	Origin (Kisanji, 1995)
Medical Educational: skills/knowledge awareness, prevention Economic Vocational Comprehensive: advocacy, legal, social, technology	Institutional Outreach Network Non-service	Professional Semi-professional Non-professionals volunteers/ persons with disabilities/ community	National/regional government Non-government – international/ national/ regional Multisectoral – international/ national/ regional Individuals – grassroots, persons with disabilities, etc.

Figure 5.1   Descriptive framework of four categories of models (adapted from McColl and Paterson, 1995).

Model 1

Aims (Murthy and Gopalan, 1992)	Structure (Peat and Boyce, 1993)	Human resources (Periquet, 1989)	Origin (Kisanji, 1995)

Medical
Educational:✓
  skill/know
  transfer✓
  awareness,
  prevention✓
Economic
Vocational
Comprehensive:
  advocacy, legal,
  social,
  technology✓
	Institutional
	Outreach
	Network
	Non-service✓
		Professional✓
		Semi-professional✓
		Non-professionals
		  volunteers/
		  persons with
		  disabilities/
		  community✓
			National/regional
			  government
			Non-government –
			  international/
			  national/
			  regional✓
			Multisectoral –
			  international/
			  national/regiona
			Individuals –
			  grassroots,
			  persons with
			  disabilities, etc.

Organization

AMREF – African Medical and Research Foundation, Community Based Rehabilitation Project in Kibwesi – Machakos District, Kenya

AMREF is an international non-government organization (NGO) based in Africa (95%) that offers a wide range of health services throughout Africa. AMREF's focus is on community based health care programmes.

Objectives

♦ Increase awareness of the need for, and importance of, early detection, intervention and prevention of disability in the community.
♦ Train teachers and community health workers in simple rehabilitation skills, knowledge and attitude, support and monitoring.
♦ Vocational training.

Activities

♦ Awareness raising and community mobilization.
♦ Community training.
♦ Use of simple appropriate technology.
♦ Establishment of community based day-care centres (playgroups).
♦ Supporting families through home visits.
♦ Arrangement of surgical intervention and follow-up activity.
♦ Institutional building of support groups.

Model 2			
Aims (Murthy and Gopalan, 1992)	Structure (Peat and Boyce, 1993)	Human resources (Periquet, 1989)	Origin (Kisanji, 1995)
Medical✓ Educational: skills/knowledge awareness, prevention✓ Economic Vocational Comprehensive: advocacy, legal, social, technology	Institutional Outreach Network✓ Non-service	Professional✓ Semi-professional Non-professionals volunteers/ persons with disabilities/ community	National/regional government Non-government – international/ national/ regional✓ Multisectoral – international/ national/regional Individuals – grassroots, persons with disabilities, etc.

Organization

Community Rehabilitation Program, Alberta

Community Rehabilitation Program is a regional rehabilitation programme, administered through the regional health authority, and funded by the Alberta Health Insurance Plan by shifting existing resources in the system to the community.

Objectives

♦ Address gaps in the current delivery of rehabilitation services.

♦ Coordinate rehabilitation with other services in acute care, long-term care, health units and private practice.
♦ Ensure that access to programme does not require physician referral.

Activities

♦ Provision of rehabilitation services at community level.
♦ Development of wellness and prevention programmes.

Model 3

Aims (Murthy and Gopalan, 1992)	Structure (Peat and Boyce, 1993)	Human resources (Periquet, 1989)	Origin (Kisanji, 1995)
Medical✓ Educational: ✓ skills/ knowledge✓ skills/ knowledge✓ Economic Vocational Comprehensive: advocacy, legal, social, technology	Institutional Outreach✓ Network✓ Non-service	Professional✓ Semi-professional✓ Non-professionals volunteers/ persons with disabilities/ community	National/regional government✓ Non-government – international/ national/regional Multisectoral – international/ national/regional Individuals – grassroots, persons with disabilities, etc.

Organization

Community Based Rehabilitation Programme at Scott Hospital, Morija, South Africa

The CBR programme was established in 1988.

Objectives

- Establish a CBR programme in the Scott Hospital Health Service Area.
- Introduce the concept of CBR to primary health care (PHC) management and staff and agree on its implementation.
- Disseminate information on CBR through orientation courses and public meetings (with chiefs and their communities).
- Raise awareness of CBR and change

- attitudes towards people with disabilities.
- Train PHC staff who will train CBR workers in the villages.
- Support and supervise training of CBR workers in the villages.
- Motivate and assist communities in the establishment of local support groups.

Activities

- Sensitization and organization of orientation courses for PHC and CBR workers.
- Integration of children with disabilities in local schools.
- Training of PHC staff and training CBR workers in the villages.
- Establishing channels of communication between CBR workers and health centre and hospital staff.

Model 4			
Aims (Murthy and Gopalan, 1992)	Structure (Peat and Boyce, 1993)	Human resources (Periquet, 1989)	Origin (Kisanji, 1995)
Medical✓	Institutional	Professional	National/regional government
Educational: ✓	Outreach	Semi-professional✓	Non-government – international/ national/regional
skills/	Network	Non-professionals	
knowledge✓	Non-service	volunteers/	
awareness,		persons with	Multisectoral – international/ national/regional
prevention✓		disabilities/	
Economic		community✓	
Vocational			Individuals – grassroots, persons with disabilities, etc.✓
Comprehensive:			
advocacy, legal,			
social, technology			

Organization

Guyana Community Based Rehabilitation Programme – Guyana

The project introduced a CBR programme to volunteers and teachers who, in turn, work with disabled children and their families.

Objectives

+ Assist the development of children with disabilities in coastal areas of Guyana.
+ Recruit and train volunteers from within the community to work with those children and their families.
+ Provide ideas and materials for the training of children with disabilities in self-help skills at community level.
+ Sensitize participants for early detection.
+ Promote community involvement in meeting the needs of people with disabilities.
+ Produce audio-visual materials locally.

Activities

+ Education of the community.
+ Recruitment and training of volunteers.
+ Formation of a Regional CBR Committee.
+ Implementation of resource units in order to create and nurture a supportive environment.

Model 5

Aims (Murthy and Gopalan, 1992)	Structure (Peat and Boyce, 1993)	Human resources (Periquet, 1989)	Origin (Kisanji, 1995)

Medical
Educational: ✓
  skills/
  knowledge✓
  awareness,
  prevention✓
Economic✓
Vocational✓
Comprehensive:
  advocacy, legal,
  social, technology
	Institutional
	Outreach
	Network✓
	Non-service
		Professional✓
		Semi-professional✓
		Non-professionals
		  volunteers/
		  persons with
		  disabilities/
		  community
			National/regional
			  government
			Non-government –
			  international/
			  national/
			  regional✓
			Multisectoral –
			  international/
			  national/regional
			Individuals –
			  grassroots,
			  persons with
			  disabilities, etc.

Organization

Union of Palestinian Medical Relief Committees (UPMRC) – West Bank and Gaza Strip, Palestine/Israel

UPMRC was established in 1979. UPMRC introduced a system of primary health care services, in order to meet the needs of rural and refugee camp communities. The programme gradually developed, from providing crucial emergency services at the community level, into a full CBR programme.

Objectives

♦ Assist people with a disability (PWD) to live independently and counsel them and their families.
♦ Facilitate their integration into the community.
♦ Facilitate education, employment and vocational training of PWD.
♦ Raise general consciousness and build awareness for both PWD and their communities at large.

Activities

♦ Establishment of community resource centres that animate several activities such as general literacy, sewing classes and vocational training.
♦ Changing the attitude of the students and teachers and integration of PWD into normal school.
♦ Helping schools in adaption to the needs of PWD.
♦ Training of community rehabilitation workers (mostly women).
♦ Provision of referral system.

Model 6			
Aims (Murthy and Gopalan, 1992)	Structure (Peat and Boyce, 1993)	Human resources (Periquet, 1989)	Origin (Kisanji, 1995)
Medical Educational: skills/knowledge awareness, prevention✓ Economic✓ Vocational✓ Comprehensive: advocacy, legal, social, technology	Institutional Outreach Network Non-service✓	Professional Semi-professional Non-professionals incl. volunteers/ persons with disabilities/ community✓	National/regional government Non-government – international/ national/regional Multisectoral – international/ national/regional Individuals – grassroots, persons with disabilities, etc.✓

Organization

Sahaya CBR Project – India

The Sahaya CBR programme was implemented by Rayalaseema Sava Samithi (RASS), an NGO established in 1981. The RASS started a CBR programme for disabled children of Tirupati and surrounding villages.

Objectives

- Make the project self-supporting through income generation programme, income to PWD and income to the project for carrying the services.
- Render comprehensive services to PWD.
- Facilitate the integration and involvement of PWD into the community life.

- Promote active participation of the community and change the attitude of the community about disability.

Activities

- Identification of the children with disabilities.
- Involvement of community leaders, youth and women representatives.
- Medical intervention by a rehabilitation institute and government hospitals.
- Integration of the physically handicapped children in the normal schools.
- Establishment of special schools.
- Marketing the items prepared by children with disabilities.

Model 7

Aims (Murthy and Gopalan, 1992)	Structure (Peat and Boyce, 1993)	Human resources (Periquet, 1989)	Origin (Kisanji, 1995)

Medical✓
Educational:
  skills/knowledge✓
  awareness,
  prevention✓
Economic✓
Vocational✓
Comprehensive:
  advocacy, legal,
  social, technology
	Institutional
	Outreach
	Network✓
	Non-service
		Professional
		Semi-professional
		Non-professionals
		  volunteer/
		  persons
		  with disabilities/
		  community✓
			National/regional
			  government
			Non-government –
			  international/
			  national/regional
			Multisectoral –
			  international/
			  national/regional
			Individuals –
			  grassroots,
			  persons with
			  disabilities, etc.✓

Organization

'SOURABHA' CBR Programme for the Disabled – India

The NGO Shree Ramana Maharishi Academy for the Blind, which had been working with visually impaired people for 25 years, moved on to fulfil the needs of all categories of people with disabilities especially in rural areas close to Bangalore. The services focus on physical and mental disabilities in the age range 0 to 50 years.

Objectives

♦ Concentrate on sustainability through building up community volunteers.
♦ Raise funds from the local community.
♦ Maximize the use of available resources from the community.

♦ Start training income generation programmes in the community.

Activities

♦ Health, medical and economic rehabilitation.
♦ Education.
♦ Awareness building.
♦ Development of curriculum and training manual for CBR workers.

Resources

♦ Professional staff members and CBR workers, trained and experienced in the field.
♦ Community volunteers.

Model 8			
Aims (Murthy and Gopalan, 1992)	Structure (Peat and Boyce, 1993)	Human resources (Periquet, 1989)	Origin (Kisanji, 1995)
Medical✓ Educational: skills/ knowledge✓ awareness, prevention✓ Economic Vocational Comprehensive: advocacy, legal, social, technology✓	Institutional Outreach✓ Network Non-service	Professional✓ Semi-professional✓ Non-professionals volunteers/ persons with disabilities/ community✓	National/regional government✓ Non-government – international/ national/regional Multisectoral – international/ national/regional Individuals – grassroots, persons with disabilities, etc.

Organization

Negros Occidental Rehabilitation Foundation (NORFI) – WHO Collaborating Center for Rehabilitation, Philippines

NORFI operates the Negros Occidental Rehabilitation Center (NORC) and manages the CBR Services (CBRS) in villages within Bacolod City and Negros Occidental. NORFI deals with cross-disability from all ages.

Objectives

+ Provide methods for disability assessments, management and referral.
+ Extend limited rehabilitation into the community through a network of trained local manpower.
+ Provide disability prevention programme at the community level.
+ Encourage PWD and their families to be part of the decision-making process.

+ Place emphasis on social integration of disabled persons.
+ Provide appropriate, affordable locally-made devices acceptable and functional in the home environment.

Activities

+ Creation of a CBRS project organization and management structure.
+ Identification and training of CBR field workers; family trainers.
+ Social preparation activities, community participation and social integration of PWD.
+ Prevention and early identification of disabilities.
+ Provision of rehabilitation services, including activities of daily living (ADL), assistive devices, referrals, sports and recreation.
+ Establishment of a referral system.

Model 9

Aims (Murthy and Gopalan, 1992)	Structure (Peat and Boyce, 1993)	Human resources (Periquet, 1989)	Origin (Kisanji, 1995)

Medical
Educational:
  skills/knowledge
  awareness,
  prevention✓
Economic
Vocational
Comprehensive:
  advocacy, legal,
  social,
  technology✓
	Institutional
	Outreach
	Network
	Non-service✓
		Professional
		Semi-professional
		Non-professionals
		  volunteers/
		  persons with
		  disabilities/
		  community✓
			National/regional
			  government
			Non-government –
			  international/
			  national/regional
			Multisectoral –
			  international/
			  national/regional
			Individuals –
			  grassroots,
			  persons with
			  disabilities, etc.✓

Organization

Persons United for Self-Help in Ontario (PUSH Ontario), Canada

PUSH Ontario is the cross-disability consumer advocate for people with disabilities in Ontario. The organization was created in 1981, when disabled consumers in Ontario began to recognize the need for groups which could advocate for civil rights of people with disabilities, such as employment, human rights, housing and transportation.

Objective

◆ Improve services to people with disabilities, to achieve integration, and to secure self-determination.

Activities

◆ Participation in coalitions, projects, the courts and independent campaigns.
◆ Advocacy activities related to issues such as transportation, employment, human rights, income maintenance, housing, long-term care and health services, substance abuse and sexuality.
◆ Organization of seminars and conferences to educate local members on issues of importance, such as employment equity, housing, drugs and disability.
◆ Education of consumers with disabilities and the wider community about disabilities.
◆ Lobbying for the workplace rights of people with disabilities.
◆ Making recommendations for the implementation of employment equity legislation as well as a series of positive measures to effectively eliminate discrimination in the workplace.

Model 10			
Aims (Murthy and Gopalan, 1992)	Structure (Peat and Boyce, 1993)	Human resources (Periquet, 1989)	Origin (Kisanji, 1995)
Medical Educational: skills/knowledge awareness, prevention Economic Vocational Comprehensive: advocacy, legal, social, technology✓	Institutional Outreach Network Non-service✓	Professional Semi-professional✓ Non-professionals volunteers/ persons with disabilities/ community✓	National/regional government✓ Non-government – international/ national/regional Multisectoral – international/ national/regional Individuals – grassroots, persons with disabilities, etc.✓

Organization

Independent Living – Kingston Independent Living Resource Center, Canada

The KILRC is a resource centre working with people with disabilities to support their efforts to live independently in the community.

Objectives

♦ Redress the imbalance in the disability world which is dominated by professionals, systems, and services.
♦ Promote and enable the progressive progress of disabled persons taking responsibilities for the development and management of personal and community resources.

♦ Be consumer controlled, community-based and cross-disability oriented.
♦ Empower PWD.
♦ Promote integration and full participation.

Activities

♦ Providing peer support and recreation.
♦ Promoting opportunities for PWD to share information, ideas, life experiences and skills.
♦ Providing information on social services and community resources and referral.
♦ Individual advocacy is akin to individual problem-solving, skill enhancement, and negotiation with services and systems in order to enhance personal resources and empowerment.

Model 11

Aims (Murthy and Gopalan, 1992)	Structure (Peat and Boyce, 1993)	Human resources (Periquet, 1989)	Origin (Kisanji, 1995)
Medical	Institutional	Professional	National/regional government
Educational: skills/knowledge awareness, prevention	Outreach Network Non-service✓	Semi-professional Non-professionals volunteers/ persons with disabilities/ community✓	Non-government – international/ national/regional
Economic Vocational✓			Multisectoral – international/ national/regional
Comprehensive: advocacy, legal, social, technology✓			Individuals – grassroots, persons with disabilities, etc.✓

Organization

Physically Challenged Farmers of Alberta, Canada

The project assists physically impaired farmers in the province to return to farm settings after injury and lead productive lives. Disabled Farmers of Alberta is a non-governmental organization operating at grassroots level.

Objectives

♦ Locate farmers with disabilities.
♦ Identify the needs of farmers with disabilities.
♦ Adapt farm equipment and farm setting to the needs of farmers with disabilities.
♦ Bring in the appropriate individuals to assist with adaptations.
♦ Assess personal care needs.
♦ Monitor progress of farmer and farm family.

Activities

♦ Identification of farmers with disabilities.
♦ Gathering and dissemination of information.
♦ Rehabilitation of farmers in order to enable them to return to farming.
♦ Assisting farmers in the process of adaptation of their environment.
♦ Publishing newsletter.

Model 12			
Aims (Murthy and Gopalan, 1992)	Structure (Peat and Boyce, 1993)	Human resources (Periquet, 1989)	Origin (Kisanji, 1995)
Medical Educational: skills/knowledge awareness, prevention Economic Vocational Comprehensive: advocacy, legal, social, technology✓	Institutional Outreach Network Non-service✓	Professional✓ Semi-professional Non-professionals volunteers/ persons with disabilities/ community✓	National/regional government Non-government – international/ national/regional Multisectoral – international/ national/regional Individuals – grassroots, persons with disabilities, etc.✓

Organization

Yee Hong Community Wellness Foundation, Scarborough, Canada

The Yee Hong Community Wellness Foundation in Scarborough is developing a support group in the Chinese–Canadian community to assist individuals and their families to adapt to changes resulting from stroke.

Objectives

♦ Develop a self sustaining Stroke Club in the Yee Hong Elderly Center, for Chinese speaking residents who have had a cerebral vascular accident.
♦ Improve effectiveness of communication between Chinese patients and non-Chinese speaking health care providers.

♦ Design and produce an information pamphlet for Chinese patients and their families.

Activities

♦ Recommending, overseeing and continuing global supervision of development, implementation and management for the stroke programme.
♦ Participation in the client and volunteer recruitment.
♦ Producing the education pamphlet in Chinese and promotion of the stroke programme.
♦ Establishing a community means of communication with a high risk group of seniors to promote wellness, activation and ongoing health screening.
♦ Integration of the Stroke Club into a nursing home environment.

Model 13

Aims (Murthy and Gopalan, 1992)	Structure (Peat and Boyce, 1993)	Human resources (Periquet, 1989)	Origin (Kisanji, 1995)
Medical✓ Educational: skills/knowledge awareness, prevention✓ Economic Vocational Comprehensive: advocacy, legal, social, technology	Institutional Outreach Network✓ Non-service	Professional✓ Semi-professional Non-professionals volunteers/ persons with disabilities/ community	National/regional government Non-government – international/ national/regional Multisectoral – international/ national/regional Individuals – grassroots, persons with disabilities, etc.✓

Organization

Community practice rehabilitation clinics (multiple examples throughout Canada)

The multidisciplinary teams of community practice rehabilitation clinics have been established to provide quick access to the assessment and treatment. They have proactive client centred approach.

Objectives

♦ Provide rehabilitation services on an outpatient basis, located in a community setting (e.g. rural village, e.g. shopping centre).

Activities

♦ Implementation of the specialized motor vehicle accident programme.
♦ Functional capacity evaluation.
♦ Implementation of osteoporosis programme.
♦ Provision of sports and orthopaedic therapy.
♦ Provision of occupational therapy.
♦ Implementation of individualized supervised exercise programmes.
♦ Education.
♦ Promotion of home exercise programmes.

Model 14			
Aims (Murthy and Gopalan, 1992)	Structure (Peat and Boyce, 1993)	Human resources (Periquet, 1989)	Origin (Kisanji, 1995)
Medical✓ Educational: skills/ knowledge✓ awareness, prevention✓ Economic Vocational Comprehensive: advocacy, legal, social, technology	Institutional Outreach✓ Network Non-service	Professional✓ Semi-professional Non-professionals volunteers/ persons with disabilities/ community	National/regional government✓ Non-government – international/ national/regional Multisectoral – international/ national/regional Individuals – grassroots, persons with disabilities, etc.

Organization

The Travelling Clinics of Newfoundland and Labrador: the Children's Rehabilitation Center

This is an institution-based programme for children with physical disabilities that services the entire province. The programme provides clinical service to patients, identifies new cases, provides education for local medical staff and community members in their own environment.

Objectives

♦ Provide necessary services to children with disabilities in their own community.

Activities

♦ Provision of individual treatment sessions, in-depth assessment and home or school visit.
♦ Identification of new cases.
♦ Education of local medical staff.
♦ Education of community members.
♦ Consultation with community workers.

Model 15

Aims (Murthy and Gopalan, 1992)	Structure (Peat and Boyce, 1993)	Human resources (Periquet, 1989)	Origin (Kisanji, 1995)

Medical✓
 Educational: ✓
   skills/knowledge
   awareness,
   prevention
 Economic
 Vocational
 Comprehensive:
   advocacy, legal,
   social, technology
	Institutional
	 Outreach✓
	 Network
	 Non-service
		Professional✓
		 Semi-professional
		 Non-professionals
		   volunteers/
		   persons with
		   disabilities/
		   community
			National/regional
			   government✓
			 Non-government –
			   international/
			   national/regional
			 Multisectoral –
			   international/
			   national/regional
			 Individuals –
			   grassroots,
			   persons with
			   disabilities, etc.

Organization

The Terry Fox Mobile Clinic: Outreach Rehabilitation in Eastern and Northeastern Ontario

The Terry Fox Mobile Clinic was established by the Rehabilitation Center, part of the Royal Ottawa Health Care Group affiliated with the University of Ottawa. It provides rehabilitation services to adults with disabilities in their own communities.

Objectives

♦ Provide consultation and resource service in specialized rehabilitation.

♦ Provide education and information resource for the community on intervention strategies and new and innovative rehabilitation procedures and technology.
♦ Evaluate the ongoing delivery of services provided and to promote development of community based health care research.

Activities

♦ Assessment and treatment of PWD in their community.
♦ Consultations.
♦ Educational sessions on various topics for PWD, families and health personnel.

Model 16

Aims (Murthy and Gopalan, 1992)	Structure (Peat and Boyce, 1993)	Human resources (Periquet, 1989)	Origin (Kisanji, 1995)
Medical✓ Educational: ✓ skills/knowledge awareness, prevention Economic Vocational Comprehensive: advocacy, legal, social, technology	Institutional Outreach Network✓ Non-service	Professional✓ Semi-professional Non-professionals✓ volunteers/ persons with disabilities/ community	National/regional government Non-government – international/ national/ regional✓ Multisectoral – international/ national/regional Individuals – grassroots, persons with disabilities, etc.

Organization

Arthritis Society Outreach Programme in British Columbia and Yukon

The national Arthritis Society established a multifaceted approach to providing care and support throughout the province to people affected by arthritis.

Objectives

♦ Provide care to those with arthritis in most communities of the province by promoting research, treatment and education.

Activities

♦ Provision of home care physiotherapy.
♦ Provision of the travelling occupational therapy service.
♦ Provision of the travelling consultation service.
♦ Implementation of the arthritis self-management programme, an education programme for patients.
♦ Implementation of the aquatic exercise programme.
♦ The outreach education programme.
♦ Development of the volunteer network.
♦ Implementation of the community based treatment programmes.

Model 17

Aims (Murthy and Gopalan, 1992)	Structure (Peat and Boyce, 1993)	Human resources (Periquet, 1989)	Origin (Kisanji, 1995)
Medical✓	Institutional	Professional✓	National/regional
Educational:	Outreach	Semi-professional✓	government
skills/knowledge	Network✓	Non-professionals	Non-government –
awareness,	Non-service	volunteers/	international/
prevention✓		persons with	national/
Economic		disabilities/	regional✓
Vocational		community	Multisectoral –
Comprehensive:			international/
advocacy, legal,			national/regional
social,			Individuals –
technology			grassroots,
			persons with
			disabilities, etc.

Organization

Community Based Vocational Rehabilitation, Ibadan, Nigeria

The community based vocational rehabilitation project in Ibadan offers income generating opportunities for people with disabilities through encouraging banks to give loans for small businesses run by PWD.

Objectives

♦ Ensure full integration of PWD into the community by providing vocational training and loan scheme for PWD in order to enable them to become economically independent and live productive lives.

Activities

♦ Organization of the vocational training.

♦ Development of income generating projects that enable PWD to earn a living from an economic activity.

♦ Involvement of local credit institutions in the loan scheme for PWD with normal interest and repayment conditions.

Model 18			
Aims (Murthy and Gopalan, 1992)	Structure (Peat and Boyce, 1993)	Human resources (Periquet, 1989)	Origin (Kisanji, 1995)
Medical✓ Educational: skills/knowledge awareness, prevention Economic Vocational Comprehensive: advocacy, legal, social, technology✓	Institutional Outreach Network✓ Non-service	Professional✓ Semi-professional Non-professionals volunteers/ persons with disabilities/ community	National/regional government Non-government – international/ national/regional Multisectoral – international/ national/regional Individuals – grassroots, persons with disabilities, etc.✓

Organization

Community Oriented Rehabilitation at the Loewenstein Hospital – Rehabilitation Center, Raanana, Israel

Community oriented rehabilitation is the integration of a rehabilitation institution with primary care, and with elements of secondary care, into one system of prevention of disablements and rehabilitation targeting the large senior population and persons with disabilities.

Objectives

♦ Provide rehabilitation to individual members of a defined community inside and outside the ordinary clinical setting of the rehabilitation institution.

♦ Identify problems of PWD and seniors.

Activities

♦ Identification of PWD and their needs.
♦ Clinical rehabilitation and outreach activities.
♦ Provision of good, comprehensive, coordinated and continuous rehabilitation on an inpatient, day-care and outpatient basis.
♦ Patient and family education including self-rehabilitation.
♦ Encouraging community participation and promoting interagency cooperation.
♦ Education and training of primary care teams.
♦ Modification of the environment.

Model 19

Aims (Murthy and Gopalan, 1992)	Structure (Peat and Boyce, 1993)	Human resources (Periquet, 1989)	Origin (Kisanji, 1995)
Medical✓ Educational: ✓ skills/knowledge awareness, prevention Economic Vocational Comprehensive: advocacy, legal, social, technology	Institutional Outreach✓ Network Non-service	Professional✓ Semi-professional Non-professionals volunteers/ persons with disabilities/ community	National/regional government Non-government – international/ national/regional Multisectoral – international/ national/regional Individuals – grassroots, persons with disabilities, etc.✓

Organization

Community Based Rehabilitation Clinics, Sarajevo, Bosnia Herzegovina

Four community clinics were established in order to bring rehabilitation services to an estimated 10 000 persons with disabilities and war injured in Sarajevo.

Objectives

+ Introduce the concept and practice of community rehabilitation and facilitate reintegration of PWDs.
+ Develop core personnel and learning resources.
+ Facilitate information exchange and personnel interactions both nationally and internationally.
+ Expand the availability of CBR services within Sarajevo.

Activities

+ Provision of accessible rehabilitation services at community level and coordination of rehabilitation activities.
+ Strengthening knowledge and skill among health care providers through seminars/educational programmes.
+ Development of relevant methods of evaluation, quality assurance and monitoring.
+ Provision of equipment for outreach and home programmes for vulnerable populations.
+ Encouraging the involvement of persons with disabilities, their families and community in the development of CBR services both in the clinics and their homes.

Model 20			
Aims (Murthy and Gopalan, 1992)	Structure (Peat and Boyce, 1993)	Human resources (Periquet, 1989)	Origin (Kisanji, 1995)
Medical✓ Educational: skills/knowledge awareness, prevention Economic Vocational Comprehensive: advocacy, legal, social, technology✓	Institutional Outreach Network✓ Non-service	Professional Semi-professional Non-professionals volunteers/ persons with disabilities/ community✓	National/regional government Non-government – international/ national/regional Multisectoral – international/ national/regional Individuals – grassroots, persons with disabilities, etc.✓

Organization

PROJIMO – Programme of Rehabilitation Organized by Disabled Youth of Western Mexico

PROJIMO Project is a rural rehabilitation programme in Western Mexico, run by persons with disabilities. They provide assistance to children with severe disabilities and their families.

Objectives

♦ Help children with disabilities and their families become more self-reliant.

♦ Provide low-cost, high quality services to poor families who cannot obtain or afford services elsewhere.

Activities

♦ Provision of wide range of rehabilitation services.
♦ Provision of equipment.
♦ Family counselling and training.
♦ Work and skills training.
♦ Brace making.
♦ Artificial limbs and wheelchair making.
♦ Special seating.
♦ Therapeutic aids.

REFERENCES

Hurley, J. Birch, S. and Eyles, J. (1992) *Information, Efficiency and Decentralization within Health Care Systems*. In CHEPA Working Paper Series No. 92–21. Hamilton, Ontario, McMaster University.

Kisanji, J. (1995) Understanding community based rehabilitation models. *CBR News* **19**: 4.

McColl, M. A. and Paterson, J. (1995) *Critical Dimensions of Community-Based Rehabilitation: Development of a Descriptive Framework for CBR. Final Report to ICACBR*. Queen's University, Kingston.

Miles, M. (1994) Community based rehabilitation information accumulation and exchange: Research notes. *CBR Symposium*. Bangalore, India.

Murthy, S. P. and Gopalan, L. (1992) *Workbook on Community-based Rehabilitation Services*. Action Aid, Bangalore, India.

NORAD Seva-in-Action (1992) *Sharing Strengths: A Workshop on Community Based Rehabilitation. Conference Proceedings*. Bangalore, India.

Peat, M. and Boyce, W. (1993) Canadian community rehabilitation services: Challenges for the future. *Canadian Journal of Rehabilitation* **6**: 281–289.

Periquet, A. O. (1989) Community-based rehabilitation in the Philippines. *International Disability Studies* **11**: 95–96.

chapter six

Planning and Management of Community Based Rehabilitation Programmes

INTRODUCTION

Persons with disabilities require a broad range of health and social programmes and services. These can range from formal programmes aimed at improving functional capacity and creating opportunities for education, vocational training, employment and legal representation, to informal activities aimed at environmental change. The success of community based rehabilitation (CBR) programmes lies in the fact that they more effectively utilize the limited financial, technological and human resources available within the community. Planning and managing are essential features in the implementa-tion and organization of CBR. These two related tools must be used effectively to design and implement programmes that are responsive to unique local and per-sonal needs, values and preferences.

CBR PROGRAMME PLANNING AND MANAGEMENT

Planning is the process of identifying the fundamental values of a community and translating them into programme priori-ties and objectives, delineating basic structures for a programme and develop-ing guidelines for the use of resources. The planning process determines such fundamental factors as the balance between the needs of the individual and those of the community, the role and relationship between institutional and community based care, the degree of integration and coordination with vocational, social, legal or educational services, and the number and distribution of human resources.

Planning models must take into account the importance of the cultural and social context of a community. CBR programmes vary within the cultural and social community framework. Planning must be done in the context of the local knowledge base, and should include key informants and stakeholders in the process. These individuals would include persons with disabilities, their families, community leader, teachers, religious leaders and politicians.

Management takes the basic system characteristics that emerge from the planning process and develops programmes to implement services or strategies in ways that are consistent with the original priorities, characteristics and objectives (Hurley et al., 1992). Management determines the organizational features of a programme, which programmes will be provided, and the relationship of a proposed programme to a greater system. Responsibility for evaluating the performance of the programmes often rests with management.

OWNERSHIP AND GOVERNANCE

A critical issue in all health and social programmes is the control of management, funding and service functions. In conventional health and social programmes, the health professions have been able to retain control of planning and decision-making processes, and have identified priorities and allocated

resources. The current trend, however, is toward the development of programmes with the objective of community ownership and operation. In health and social programmes offered by government or non-government sponsored agencies, power frequently remains with those who control finances and resource allocation. Although in many instances alternative governance structures can create a perception of independence, donor agencies may exert influence which can override the opinions and recommendations of the participants. An essential feature of management in CBR is shared responsibility and true and equal partnership.

The traditional employer/employee management relationship has been less successful when applied to community development programmes. Partnership is critical when CBR programmes are first initiated and professionals and volunteers are seeking the most appropriate entry point into a community. Community participation facilitates general acceptance and encourages collaboration and commitment. Organizations of persons with disabilities are critical of agencies that are unwilling to work on a full partnership basis. As a result there are examples of successful CBR programmes which were initiated by non-professionals and community individuals or groups, in a format which minimizes or eliminates participation by health professionals.

Ownership and governance issues in community development are areas of great sensitivity. Community development programmes, whether dealing with disability or development issues, must emphasize the application of strategies which truly reflect the skills and commitment of all participants and stakeholders. Vulnerable populations, such as persons with disabilities and women, have traditionally been under-represented, particularly in governance and management strategies.

DECENTRALIZATION AND COMMUNITY BASED REHABILITATION

One of the key features of CBR programmes is decentralization, the shifting of planning, management and decision-making to local levels. Decentralization, particularly with respect to planning and management, is commonly viewed as a means of making health and social programmes more responsive to local needs, values and preferences (Peat, 1991).

In its 1978 declaration *Health for All*, the World Health Organization identified district level planning as the key to developing primary care centred health systems (WHO, 1981). In recent years a number of countries have either implemented, or are trying to implement, varying degrees of decentralization. For instance, New Zealand has created area health boards with broad responsibilities for health care services for geographically defined populations. In Canada, a number of provincial commissions (Nova Scotia, Saskatchewan, Ontario and British Columbia) have called for further decentralization while some provinces (Alberta, Quebec) have implemented local area health boards. Although there are many different definitions of decentralization, all seem to agree that decentralization means shifting the locus of decision-making power to local or regional levels which increases their autonomy and scope for independent action (Hurley *et al.*, 1992). Decentralization increases public participation in decision-making and the accountability to the public of planners, managers and providers.

Although decentralization and decision-making at the community level are essential features for successful CBR programmes, it is important that decentralization does not create a sense of isolation.

The management of CBR must interface effectively with other community services and programmes which provide the broad spectrum of resources required by persons with disabilities and their families. Often it is assumed that decentralization translates into local democracy, but this is not always the case. In various parts of the world, most notably in rural communities, some local leaders exercise a high degree of social control (Helander, 1993). To avoid a monopoly of power, CBR programmes must create planning and management processes that encourage community participation. The progressive CBR community is one that has existing traditions of involving citizens in the decision-making process.

MANAGEMENT OF COMMUNITY BASED REHABILITATION PROGRAMMES

One of the first considerations in an approach to CBR is to be sensitive to, and learn from, the people. Community based rehabilitation is first and foremost 'community'. Learning from the community, from the successes and failures of other programmes and from the creative and innovative training and copying that occurs spontaneously as people deal with issues of common concern, is of vital importance to any planner. As communities are already organized, planning and management techniques are already being employed in the community setting. CBR programme management must learn from, and respect, the local environment in order to meet the needs of the person with a disability within their own social and cultural context.

Planners and managers are discouraged from applying preset programme models or standardized systems imported from other communities. There are programme aspects that may be duplicated, and there is valuable learning that can take place from the experiences of others, but each initiative must be unique to the community it serves and adapted to each unique cultural environment. Local planners and managers, by virtue of being closer to, and more familiar with, the communities in which they serve, may be able to accrue additional information not available to planners and policy-makers who are removed from the local situation, particularly knowledge regarding needs, values and preferences. A local manager has more knowledge of the skills of local workers, and a better sense of how technology will fit, where and how people live, and the needs of the people – all of which contribute to a more effective programme design.

Strategic Planning

Once it has been established that a community initiative will be undertaken, and the community has indicated its needs and willingness to commit human and structural resources, then it is important that the community understands how these translate into a plan for action. The details of the expected outcome of a CBR programme should be discussed and documented in a strategic planning process. If the programme deals with rehabilitation service delivery, then this process should detail whether or not central health care institutions will be accessed, what external support is available from the central stytem, what local resources are currently available and still need to be mobilized for training and technical supervision, and how referrals will be managed.

General involvement of the community stakeholders in the programme's strategic planning process is necessary so that common goals, interests and understanding may be developed prior to programme development and implementation. The mission statement and proposed goals and objectives of the programme should be clearly stated and broadly circulated within the community.

Structure and Organization

It is very difficult to design a decision-making structure that represents community interests while at the same time integrating them with expert knowledge in a balanced manner. Management structure should reflect a philosophy of sharing, consulting, negotiation and decision-making or veto power. A central aspect of CBR is the concept of actively involving persons with disabilities and their families in the planning and implementation of programmes.

A common approach to the planning and management of CBR is the use of a 'board' or 'committee'. Members may be elected or appointed, and often include persons with disabilities, family members, professionals, representatives of local organizations such as women's groups and businesses, and influential leaders such as the school principal, the head of a religious group or a local political figure such as the mayor. Other important members who might be considered for membership on a committee or board would be a representative of the local organization for people with disabilities or family support group (Helander, 1993). In order to be properly accountable for themselves, community boards need to develop a strong sense of their role in the process of CBR and what and whom they are representing.

A CBR committee may be struck to conduct all, or some, of the management functions. Typical tasks of the committee might include:

- planning and organizing the development of the CBR programme: selecting community rehabilitation workers, volunteers and other staff; defining roles and tasks for participants;
- managing operations of the CBR programme: controlling, tracking, documenting and reporting financial information; reviewing, reporting and monitoring information;
- organizing community awareness activities that fit with community attitudes toward disability and the CBR programme and identifying key issues for discussion;
- influencing resource mobilization by selecting the most appropriate fundraising activities.

Programme Roles and Responsibilities

I think that if CBR could be developed in a direction where, from the start, disabled people, and their leaders are actively involved in planning, implementing and monitoring the process, the results could be better and more lasting. (Konkkola, 1990).

Community development programmes involve active participation of individuals and groups representative of the social, cultural and economic nature of society. In the development of roles and responsibilities, the first priority is to ensure that there is involvement of persons with disabilities in all aspects and roles of the programmes.

The roles and responsibilities of CBR personnel will be determined by the nature of the community and society in which the CBR programme is located and may vary considerably depending upon whether the programme occurs in a rural community in an economically disadvantaged society or an urban community in an economically advantaged environment. The following are examples of common roles in CBR programmes, the applicability and relevance will therefore depend on the nature of the programme itself.

Trainers

Basic-level services can be delivered by 'trainers'. These may be volunteers, and/or persons with disabilities themselves or their families who may receive training and supervision from community workers. The basic level of service provision within the community can be provided in a variety of ways. Some workers assume this role parallel to other employment, and in some cases, the community provides compensation to make the activity a full-time occupation. A community worker, after receiving training and successfully filling the role, may progress to the position of CBR local supervisor.

Community Workers

The community worker must be highly motivated and literate. Local supervisors or community workers are trained and supervised by professionals or multidisciplinary resource teachers. Community workers are often responsible for contacting local resource persons and agencies to assist persons with disabilities find services which provide vocational training and employment assistance. Community trainers provide basic instruction and supervision of family members or 'trainers' regarding the action to be taken. Problems that cannot be solved at this level would be referred to another level of the system, or in the case of health care services, to the rehabilitation professional. In some countries the supervisor is a volunteer; in others, some compensation, not necessarily a salary, is needed (Helander, 1993).

Functions of community workers include:

♦ disability identification, location of persons with disabilities;
♦ helping people with disabilities and their families to assess progress and needs;
♦ giving simple non-professional assistance, advice and support;
♦ making appropriate referrals to a specialist or agencies;
♦ helping with, or leading community training and education.

Intermediate Level Community Supervisor

An intermediate level community supervisor could be a nurse, therapist, teacher or a person with a disability, or community worker who has proved capable and will fulfil this function where there are a number of related CBR activities or programmes which require overall coordination and management.

Volunteers

There are several different classifications or groups of volunteers.

♦ persons with disabilities themselves;
♦ family members of persons with disabilities;
♦ community workers, recruited from the community;
♦ school teachers, not necessarily with special training;
♦ members of the community at large;
♦ members of community organizations;
♦ persons at all levels of government, political leaders, local authorities, religious leaders.

To volunteer does not necessarily mean that people work without any reward, compensation or recognition. Locally recruited volunteers normally have a stronger sense of community, and families of persons with disabilities or persons with disabilities themselves are strongly motivated to contribute voluntarily. Non-monetary forms of compensation can include various forms of appreciation and esteem from the community. In some developing societies, volunteering leads to permanent employment. In some societies, volunteering can also give social acceptance for women to function outside of the traditional family unit. Family members who volunteer are rewarded with the developing independence of the disabled family member (Lysack and Krefting, 1993).

Professionals

The conventional health care and social service delivery model has been shown to be one where clinical expertise and knowledge are owned by the practitioner and employed in a highly technological, specialized institutional setting. As health care delivery shifts to a community focus, the role of the professional changes to that of observer, counsellor, fact finder, collaborative problem solver, information specialist and advocate (Pickles, 1989). In other words, the role of the professional is to inspire and to encourage communities to find their own solutions and build up their own resources and experiences.

Full-time Professionals

Where professionals have a full-time function in a CBR programme, there is often significant ownership of the programme by government or non-government agencies external to the community itself. In societies where the number of health professionals is limited or inadequate, greater opportunities exist for professionals to define their own roles in community progammes and assume responsibilities that are not normally associated with their roles in institutional programmes. If there is only one health professional in a community development programme, the opportunity to function on a one-to-one basis with persons with disabilities would be limited. In this situation, the professional is more likely to become a manager or organizer responsible for programme design, evaluation and training functions.

Part-time Professionals

Part-time involvement in community development programmes has been traditionally the most common form of professional participation, particularly in developing societies. Part-time commitment can be occasional, periodic, limited assignment or preparatory and may occur regularly by week, day or on a sporadic basis. The role of part-time professionals in CBR development is of importance as it is frequently the only link between a community programme and the essential knowledge base. Many non-government programmes have developed CBR with a limited degree of professional involvement.

Performance Evaluation

Performance areas may overlap within the training and management of staff and volunteers. From management's point of view, day-to-day performance evaluation is a process that determines the degree of success in achieving predetermined objectives. If the objectives are defined in a job description, then performance can be measured against known and agreed upon standards. A performance appraisal is also an effective means of identifying the particular training and

developmental needs of individual participants in a CBR activity.

Day-to-day performance evaluation over a given period of time gives the employees or volunteers an opportunity to express concerns, ideas, personal goals and ambitions. Feedback on performance can be a significant motivator for positive behavioural change. It has often been suggested that the best strategy for motivation is to provide the employee or volunteer with immediate positive feedback during the course of job duties, instead of waiting for performance evaluation on a monthly, semiannual or annual basis.

It is essential that all members of a CBR activity are involved in the process of developing and establishing their own duties and responsibilities or job description. Management must function in partnership with the employee/volunteer constituency in order to ensure that all members of the CBR process are fully supportive of their assigned responsibilities. Also, it is critical that all members of the team understand the decision-making procedures which are appropriate to the operational requirements of the programme such as hiring practices, allocation of financial resources and identification of priority areas. A performance appraisal should be regarded as an integral element of all activities and when carried out properly should be perceived as a positive and productive process.

Physical Resources

The management processes of a CBR activity must clearly identify the physical resource requirements together with the financial and personnel needs necessary for day-to-day programme activities. Sustainability is key to the success of all CBR. The planning and management processes, therefore, must develop a strategic planning framework which will accurately identify the financial and physical resources required for programme stability. The physical resource requirements of a CBR programme will depend on the nature of the programme and the scope of activities. There are many approaches to the development and implementation of CBR activities; therefore there is no 'blueprint' for a typical CBR programme and the physical resources required.

Local Structures

These resources can range from a CBR 'Centre' with evaluation, education and training programmes, clinical and counselling services each with identifiable physical resource requirements, to grassroots organizations with no formal central facility. CBR frequently occurs without the need for special buildings as programmes can take place in homes, collective housing projects, in community open-air meeting places or community buildings.

Indigenous Resources

Programme management should be aware of any local indigenous resources that could contribute to programme activities. For example, local technical facilities such as a bicycle part manufacturer could be accessed in the development of appropriate technical aids and services. An understanding and appreciation of the use of local materials and products in building design must be matched with a knowledge of local cultural, social and economic values and customs. There are examples of CBR centres being built in rural areas using building design features copied from economically advantaged urban societies. In these instances, community support and compliance has been minimal, making it virtually impossible for the CBR centre to be fully incorporated into community life.

Public Information and Policies

Management must be aware of current policy documents, regulations, legislation and public information related to the nature of any contemplated CBR activity. For example, existing public domain survey data that is available on the demographics and nature of disability will be of great value. There are many areas in which existing material and data can provide invaluable resource information relating to:

♦ local transportation systems and facilities;
♦ public information and database on persons with disabilities;
♦ government and non-government concessions and subsidies;
♦ employment regulations.

Education and Training

One of the most important aspects of CBR is education and training. In order to build competencies at the community level, a substantial investment needs to be made in education and training. Training basics would include the essential knowledge base incorporating an understanding of disability, rehabilitation strategies, communication skills and community development.

The strategic plan should identify how managerial training will be provided within the CBR programme. The management structure should include persons with disabilities and their families, many of whom will provide invaluable insight into training requirements and expected outcomes. Training and education is a critical issue to CBR and is discussed in detail in Chapter 8.

Rehabilitation Skill and Knowledge Transfer

Within the health and social disciplines, the knowledge base is considered to be the 'property' of a particular group, not to be accessed or used by other groups or individuals external to the professional discipline itself. In community development where manpower is very limited, considerable debate surrounds the issue of the sharing of knowledge and skills. Professional groups have frequently expressed considerable reservation concerning the diffusion of knowledge and skill between professions and from professionals to non-professionals. Many community development programmes would not have been possible, however, without a deliberate and active transfer of knowledge from health professionals to intermediaries or community workers. It has been argued that the dilution of the essential knowledge base can be counterproductive if it leads to inappropriate and ineffective project management and operation and a diminished quality of service. The limitations of skill and knowledge transfer must be considered within the strategic planning framework.

A further issue is the degree to which rehabilitation skill transfer should concentrate on specific technical skills without addressing the need to provide scientific information and the underlying background related to the skill itself. As a consequence, many of the techniques used to disseminate knowledge and skills are presented as a 'hands on' learning experience and have focused on a particular aspect of disability identification or management. The limitations of this experience should be understood by the management personnel who need to be aware of the advantages, disadvantages and limitations of the skill being transferred.

Finances and Funding

Origin of Programme Support

The management process must clearly identify the ongoing sources of financial support for programme activities. The essential elements of budget management and control should be identified within the strategic planning framework. The history of CBR has shown that sources of funding can range from occasional contributions to regular and predictable financial support. In a time of diminishing resources management has had to be increasingly aware of fundraising and cost-sharing strategies. The sustainability of programmes is in question where management fails to develop a financial plan and a strategy appropriate to the goals and expectations of the programme.

Financial support for CBR activities can fall into one, or any combination of the following:

- *Direct government funded*. This is seen where a national or regional government has accepted responsibility for the financial support of programme activities and the resources flow directly to CBR initiatives. An example of this funding model is the District Rehabilitation Centre Program in India.
- *Indirect government funded*. This occurs where government resources are directed through an intermediary organization. In this instance financial support is provided to a non-government organization which in turn applies the resources to a CBR programme. An example of this funding model is the financial support from international funding agencies that is provided to the Voluntary Health Services Society (VHSS) in Bangladesh, which is then allocated by VHSS to support the development of national CBR activities.

- **Non-government (non-profit, reinvested profit, self-sustaining)**. CBR in many societies has been largely dependent upon self-supporting non-government organizations. These organizations and agencies have had to develop an effective fundraising strategy in order to achieve a measure of sustainability. These organizations are vulnerable, particularly at this time of increasing competition for financial support. Sustainability in these instances is often determined by the degree to which CBR has become a community priority with commitment and ownership of the project by the community itself. Examples of this type of funding of a non-government organization are the Seva-in-Action Production and Training Centre in Bangalore, India, where low cost, culturally appropriate aids and appliances are manufactured, and the Disabled Farmers of Alberta, Canada, which assists impaired farmers in that province to return to farm settings after injury.
- **Income or profit generating**. Community development programmes linking disability issues to income generation have been a strategy which has advanced the participation of disabled persons in community life while offering opportunities for economic independence. Examples of this kind of initiative are the Pragathi Creations, Seva-in-Action programme in Bangalore, India, which is a garment factory offering training and employment to persons with disability, and the Silent World Craft, Bangkok, which produces wooden handicrafts and employs and trains persons with hearing impairment.
- **Voluntary**. There are many local community initiatives which are organized and sustained on an entirely voluntary basis. Many are uniquely local initiatives resulting from the interest of disabled persons, family members and community members. These activities are often centred around one disability issue such as poliomyelitis or cerebral palsy. In situations where a community has been greatly disadvantaged by conflict, volunteer programmes may be the only approach to CBR. The development of community programmes for the disabled in Sarajevo during the recent period of extreme hostilities was the result of local volunteer initiatives with no access to financial or other resources (Nelson *et al.*, 1994).

CBR Project Financial Management

Management must employ basic, standard and reliable financial systems to monitor, track and control expenditures. The CBR Budget Framework illustrated in Figure 6.1 is a general accounting system frequently used by managers and administrators. The operating or recurrent costs listed in this illustration are those costs that are ongoing and paid regularly. Examples of operating costs might include rent, staff wages and continuing education. Capital costs include the actual funds needed to buy particular items such as reference books, training manuals, motor vehicles and ramps. Usually capital costs are 'one time costs' and do not recur. Start-up costs cover items such as expenses incurred by the programme during the initial period of implementation including the cost of intensive initial training, renovations and public relations.

One of the organizing principles of CBR is local community ownership, therefore recording and tracking local donations of time, goods and material is an essential aspect of the monitoring and evaluation process. This information is particularly important when embarking on fundraising activities. When a programme can demonstrate in tangible terms that the community is motivated and is making a contribution, outside donors are more likely to see the programme as worthy of supplemental support. Simple data

Category	Annual cost	Percentage of total cost
Capital costs		
Equipment (computers, fax, typewriters) Vehicles (cars, motorcycles, bicycles) Building (if buying)		
One time start-up costs		
Posters, advertisements, brochures Official opening event		
Operating costs		
Staff Supplies Vehicle (operation and maintenance) Building (rent) Training (ongoing) Community meetings		

Figure 6.1 CBR budget framework.

collection should be initiated early in the programme development process. As many of the contributions are of a voluntary nature with no direct remuneration, it is important to calculate the value of the activity or resource provided. This calculation can be referred to as 'in-kind' contributions for which a cost factor should be identified and recorded. In this way the real financial value of voluntary activities is clearly identified.

In kind contributions can include:

♦ food: based on the cost if purchased in a store;
♦ donated rooms/buildings: based on the cost if rented;
♦ volunteer time: based on an average hourly wage;
♦ materials/equipment ramp, wheel-

chairs, etc.: based on the cost if purchased;
♦ donated professional time: based on actual rates or schedules;
♦ donated media coverage: based on actual fees for commercials.

Local management should ensure that this very important type of information is recorded, so that once a comprehensive evaluation review is initiated or if a sudden need for evaluation becomes evident, the information is at hand. Once the data monitoring has been set in motion, the information and techniques grow rapidly.

Community Based Rehabilitation Technology[1]

Technology is one important aspect of a community rehabilitation programme.

---

[1] An excellent resource for information on rehabilitation technology is the *Rehabilitation Technology in CBR: A Compendium* published by the International Centre for the Advancement of Community Based Rehabilitation, Kingston, Ontario, Canada K7L 3N6 (e-mail address olneys@qucdn.queensu.ca). The material in the sections on CBR technology and appropriate technology are adapted from this *Compendium*.

Assistive devices contribute to the overall objective of rehabilitation by restoring or improving a user's physical or occupational function and thereby offering a better quality of life. Under the institutional rehabilitation service model, rehabilitation technology is under the control of professionals and institutions which are often remote from the people in need. Under the CBR approach, the management and control of technology needs and services can become an important component of a CBR programme. The community programme can become the location of assessment, design, fabrication, maintenance, evaluation and training (*Compendium*, 1995).

The control and management issues related to technology which need to be addressed include:

♦ What are the priorities for fabrication, distribution, and training?
♦ What is produced?
♦ What technologies will be produced?
♦ Who receives them and what governs priority?
♦ How much do they cost and who pays for them?
♦ What mechanisms are used for assessment, distribution, servicing and education?

Specialized skills are needed in all phases of technology design, manufacture and application. The development of CBR will depend not only on the degree to which simple skills, such as metal and plastic fabrication and plaster casting, can be passed on to members of the community, but on the degree to which health care workers are willing and able to transfer their skills in evaluation and training. Professionals working in CBR must have access to the knowledge base of technological aids and devices and must be prepared to consult with the community in a flexible manner. It is important that professionals understand the needs and priorities of the individual and the community and be willing to work with community members in developing possible solutions to these identified needs and problems.

Appropriate Technology

Appropriate technology originated as a general socioeconomic ideology which was gradually applied to health care and then to rehabilitation technology. Organizations which have focused on issues related to appropriate technology include Appropriate Health Resources and Technologies Action Group (AHRTAG) and the Faculty of Appropriate Technology at the University of Eindhoven in the Netherlands. These organizations have significantly advanced the understanding of the need to design and produce technology specific to the social, economic and cultrual context of a community.

Appropriate technology in CBR programmes has included the design and development of low cost crutches, walking aids, mobility devices including wheelchairs, footwear and calipers. The organization and management of CBR programmes in which appropriate technology is an important feature must address the assessment of individual need and issues surrounding fabrication, distribution, service delivery, training of fabricators and other individuals to provide service, and the evaluation of effectiveness. Managers and designers must have an understanding of the lives, goals and special needs of consumers with a disability in developing technology which will impact on the lives of persons with disabilities. Scherer (1993) published the direct personal expressions of persons with a disability and their experiences, both positive and negative, regarding the use of assistive technology.

Prosthetics

Prosthetics is the field of knowledge concerned with the replacement of missing or removed body parts. Prostheses resemble missing body parts such as the foot, lower leg, arm, hand and joints lost through disease or accident. CBR literature deals mostly with lower limb prosthetics and the difficulty of introducing high technology prosthetics in developing countries due to the complexity of their fabrication and the extensive technical training required. The literature also demonstrates the innovative use of indigenous materials such as cane and bamboo. The development of the Jaipur foot, made of vulcanized rubber, is an excellent illustration of successful prosthetic design.

Orthotics

Orthoses are appliances for mobile parts of the body, such as limbs and the head, which might require support and stabilization. Persons use orthoses to strengthen, improve or restore function. Calipers, splints and other supports fall into this device category. CBR programmes which might involve the provision of orthotics include programmes for impairments caused by leprosy, cerebral palsy, poliomyelitis and stroke. Like prosthetics, it is important to incorporate the local, cultural and social values of users in the design process. For example, Western designs of lower limb orthoses use a shoe as the foundation of the device. This is inappropriate in cultures which requires easy removal of the shoe before entering home or places of worship or where significant ankle flexibility is required for squatting.

Activities of Daily Living (ADL)

Aids for activities of daily living are synonymous with self-help devices for use in the home. The principle behind ADL is compatible with the goals of CBR because it promotes and improves the quality of daily life for persons with a disability. These devices are designed and constructed with the user's independence and specific needs in mind, including feeding, dressing, toileting, bathing and transferring.

Mobility

Mobility is a major issue in CBR as it provides greater opportunity for education, employment, independence and self-determination. Factors controlling mobility include the extent of the area in which a person wishes to be mobile, the condition and adaptability of that area and the general physical capacity and type of disability. Different types of impairment require different types of mobility devices.[2] Paraplegics and quadriplegics may be assisted by wheeled devices such as wheelchairs and tricycles. For those without access to a wheelchair or its related technology, wheeled carts and trolleys have been fabricated.

Factors Affecting Technology in CBR

Factors that affect the development of assistive devices include:

♦ *Assessment* – the needs of the individual, evaluation of the outcome.
♦ *Design* – the conceptual leap between assessment and fabrication.

---

[2] There is a significant body of literature on wheeled mobility devices. The following merit special mention: (1) Two manuals by AHRTAG in the UK: *Personal Transport for Disabled People* by Ayre (1984) and *How to Make Simple Disability Aids* by Caston (1987), and (2) A Clinical Supplement of the *Journal of Rehabilitation Research and Development* (1992).

- *Fabrication* – use of local material and local human resources, and costs.
- *Maintenance* – user maintained.
- *Training* – users, families and local personnel in device purpose and application.
- *Evaluation* – based on general experience and observation, formal research studies.

Reporting, Monitoring and Evaluation

The monitoring of information in CBR activities must be simple and relevant. Collection of information should be part of the daily routine and should be recorded and quantified. Data collection could include numbers of people in a particular programme, how often the programmes run, how long programmes last and the specific costs of operation. Human resource data may include the number of workers, hours of paid and unpaid work, worker appointments and separations.

Programme activities may be tracked by collecting:

- the range and average number of contact hours per community worker per month;
- the number of people on waiting lists;
- the number and category of people referred;
- the percentage of time that the community worker spends providing technical aids, direct help, training the person with a disability and family and coordinating referrals.

Information collected becomes a tool for project evaluation. How and when information is collected relates to the evaluation process being undertaken.

Evaluation in CBR programmes is a topic which is dealt with in depth in Chapter 7.

PROGRAMME SUSTAINABILITY

One of the most important issues in CBR is sustainability. Whether or not a programme continues depends on the extent to which it is accepted and supported by the community. The support may come through a variety of different avenues including personnel, buildings, financial resources and day-to-day operating requirements.

One of the major functions of management is to develop the strategies which will ensure long-term viability. A major concern to all CBR programmes is the ongoing need to generate financial resources appropriate to the scale of operations so that the financial plan will balance revenue and expenditures. Where the revenue base is uncertain, the programme is continually vulnerable. In those instances where the community is the primary source of support, a significant gap between revenue and expenditure will likely lead to concerns about the programme's viability in the future.

Sustainability is not only influenced by the financial base of a CBR programme, it is also dependent on:

- effective management;
- development of a Strategic Plan;
- identification of programme objectives;
- involvement of the community;
- a plan and time line for operations;
- programme evaluation;
- the relevance of the programme to the needs of the community and regional and national priorities.

A CBR project which is not related to a government policy or programme, it has been suggested, has little chance of being sustained. Sometimes an organization in its zeal to promote CBR provides a great deal of external support to a CBR project, which is not linked to government policies or priorities. There may be a perceived need, and the community may be enthusiastic because of the initial external support. However, as the support gradually decreases the CBR project will wither and die (ILO, UNESCO, WHO, 1994).

External Sustainability

External sustainability occurs where the community initiative is supported by predictable, reliable and continuing funding sources outside the community itself. Financial, personnel and other resources may be provided as regular allocations from a sponsoring agency. This type of external sustainability creates a climate of uncertainty in that the 'client' community is vulnerable to the changing priorities of the sponsor. Sponsor funds may be provided either as 'block funding' support or on a graduated scale decreasing over an identified time. Where international agencies have provided initial funding for the development of CBR programmes, they will frequently provide the support in a time-limited manner. When sponsor funds are no longer available the community project has to become fully self-sustaining.

Community development projects frequently are terminated because of the withdrawal of financial support from the original sponsor. This may be due to changing financial priorities, unanticipated limitation of funding sources, or a philosophical change on the part of the agency or sponsor. Current trends indicate that the sustainability issue is a critical factor in all community development pro-

grammes, and one that all participants should be fully sensitive to in the design and implementation process.

Internal Sustainability

Internal sustainability of a programme occurs where financial, human and other resources are generated by the programme participants themselves with little or no reliance on, or support from, external sources. Although it may dictate a more cautious or conservative approach to development, it decreases the vulnerability of the community initiative. Frequently the strategy for sustainability of programmes will be a mix, or balance, between internal and external resources. The function of management, however, is to identify clearly what resources are required and to develop the strategies appropriate to a programme.

COMMUNICATION AND COORDINATION

In the process of planning and prior to implementing any CBR programme, a function of management would be to take an inventory of all existing systems, programmes and peripheral networks already active in the community. These might include religious leaders, teachers and educators, health workers, social service workers, staff in development programmes, social security agencies, organizations for the disabled, employment and legal aid systems (Helander, 1993).

Coordination should be aimed at economizing resources at all levels of CBR programmes. There is a need to cooperate in order to avoid duplication of services, to distribute them equitably especially to rural environments, and to share the use of cost intensive resources, professional personnel, equipment, transportation and communication. It is vital that CBR programmes communicate with each other in order to share information regarding strategies, failures and successes. The CBR environment has been faced with the difficulty of developing effective communication systems in order to share experiences. The environment of institutional rehabilitation, on the other hand, has developed a system of publishing and sharing results within the broader health science and academic and professional communities. Health science libraries internationally are major repositories of information regarding rehabilitation programmes, research and policy. The non-government organization (NGO) community within which CBR has developed, has not had access to this traditional academic communication process. However, many of the NGO agencies publish material describing the extent of their CBR initiatives such as the AHRTAG[3] and the Action Aid[4] publications.

Access to the worldwide Internet is increasingly available and the most popular Internet application, e-mail, is an electronic messaging system that enables users to send on-screen letters and documents anywhere in the world. Those seeking reference information have access to a wide variety of resources including connections to:

♦ computerized libraries;
♦ universities;
♦ government agencies;
♦ commercial and special interests groups;
♦ non-government organizations and multilateral agencies.

Recently, there have been important developments in the application of the worldwide web (www). This is a part of the Internet that links computers throughout the world through 'home pages'. This system uses pictures, graphics and sound to relay information instantly. The following are examples of home page web addresses for specific disability groups:

♦ Vocational Rehabilitation (http://www/icdi.wvu.edu);
♦ Advocacy on Special Education (http://earthlink.net/free/edlawman/web-docs);
♦ Disability Resources (http: //wideopen.igc.apr.org/pwd/disabilities.html).

GLADNET is a global effort involving the International Labour Organization (ILO) and research centres around the world. The GLADNET initiative is a result of the ILO promoting the concept of collaboration internationally, and bringing together researchers with common interests in disability (e-mail: frehab@hq111.ilo.ch). The system aims to:

♦ enhance the knowledge base on employment, training, workplace measures, return to work strategies and special needs;
♦ pool research capacities to support policies that give disabled persons equal access to labour markets;
♦ support practical and low cost solutions by sharing resources.

---

[3] Appropriate Health Resources and Technologies Action Group (AHRTAG), London, UK, produces *CBR News*.
[4] Action Aid Disability Division, PO Box 5406, 3 Rest House Road, Bangalore 560 001, India, which produces *Action Aid News*.

COMMUNITY PARTICIPATION, MOBILIZATION AND AWARENESS

The term mobilization refers to the ways in which communities are involved and encouraged to participate in CBR. CBR programmes often begin with an information campaign which encourages mobilization based on real and achievable goals and objectives, directed at clearly identified issues. Community initiative, energy and social dynamics leads to the initiation and implementation of a successful CBR programme.

The response and enthusiasm generated for the concept of CBR is strongly influenced by cultural and traditional factors. Persons with disabilities themselves can be instrumental in initiating and maintaining momentum for recognition. The process of mobilizing a community is not something that can occur overnight and it may take some time to inspire, inform and sensitize people. People in general are hesitant or careful about anything new until it can be proven to be reliable and productive. CBR may not be foremost on the minds of the community when they analyse their global community needs. However, there is always the opportunity to lay the groundwork at the level of awareness building and health promotion.

From the outset, people in communities need basic CBR information. They need to be made aware that:

♦ disability is common (although to some extent hidden);
♦ there are simple methods of training and educating people with disabilities that can take place where they live which can lead to more independence and social integration;
♦ they do not have to wait for external initiatives or the opening of institu-

tions in order to achieve some degree of health and social service in their community using an action programme of their own;
♦ there will be a community obligation to provide some resources; and
♦ there will be an expectation that the community contributes to planning, management and evaluation processes (Helander, 1993).

Information is a powerful tool for educating the community and influencing people, for preparing the way for community development and making change. Ways of using information to reach people would include:

♦ publications;
♦ special speakers, especially speakers with a disability;
♦ conferences;
♦ connections with other CBR programmes;
♦ attention to spontaneous feedback or informal feedback sessions;
♦ research;
♦ training programmes and workshops.

In many cultures, the power in the community lies with the male dominated leadership while those who actually 'do the work' are women. It is of great value for a programme to be accepted at the grassroots level by women caregivers and in the women's community groups. This basic level support base may be developed as a community entry strategy.

If a community has had previous exposure to a 'Western' medical model health care service, community members may expect CBR services to be provided in a similar manner. The CBR management should address this issue in order to prevent unreasonable expectations.

An explanation of what the term 'community' means in the term CBR and a more detailed discussion of community participation can be found in Chapter 3.

CBR PROGRAMME INFLUENCE ON PROMOTING AND DEVELOPING PUBLIC POLICIES

It has been suggested that successful CBR programmes are those that align closely with government policies (Helander, 1993). Once programmes have been established, one or a group of individuals may wish to work with government officers to effect change to policies, or assist in developing policies where none currently exist. It is important that the management of a CBR programme develop an effective relationship with those responsible for the development of public policy. Helander suggests that it is important to convince governments to modify policies and emphasizes the cost benefits of the CBR approach in his argument for change.

In summary, participatory planning and management processes and structures must be crafted to fit the particular needs of the community. The details of the expected outcomes of the CBR programme should be discussed and documented in a strategic planning process. The components of the programme should be documented, clearly stated, and given wide distribution. The programme's strategic plan should outline a simple data collection process that will form the basis for the programme's information system. The information collected should be easy to acquire without outside help. Monitoring and trend analysis should be a continuous process aimed at correcting and improving action in order to render activities more relevant, more efficient and more effective.

REFERENCES

Konkkola, K. (1990) Community based rehabilitation and independent living. *One in Ten* **8**: Issue 104, **9**: Issues 1–2.

Helander, E. (1993) *Prejudice and Dignity: An Introduction to Community Based Rehabilitation.* United Nations Development Program, New York.

Hurley, J., Birch, S. and Eyles, J. (1992) Information, efficiency and decentralization within health care systems. In *CHEPA Working Paper Series No. 92–21.* Hamilton, Ontario, Master University.

International Labour Organization (ILO), UNESCO, and the World Health Organization (WHO) (1994) *Joint Position Paper on Community Based Rehabilitation for and with People with Disabilities.* Geneva.

Lysack, C. and Krefting L. (1993) Community based rehabilitation cadres: their motivation for volunteerism. *International Journal of Rehabilitation Research* **16**: 133–141.

Nelson, M., Phripp, T., Pinkerton, C., Wangda, A. and Wangda J. (1994) *Community Based Rehabilitation: Demonstration Models.* Unpublished paper for MSc. Rehabilitation Science Course 877. Queen's University, Kingston, Canada.

Olney, S., Packer, T., Wyss, U. and Roche, J. (Eds) (1995) *A Compendium: Rehabilitation Technology in Community Based Rehabilitation.* International Centre for the Advancement of Community Based Rehabilitation. Queen's University, Kingston, Canada.

Peat, M. (1991) Community based rehabilitation: development and structure, Part 2. *Clinical Rehabilitation* **5**: 231–239.

Pickles, B. (1989) Education in community-based rehabilitation. In *Community Based Rehabilitation: International Perspectives* (conference mongraph). Queen's University, Kingston, Canada.

Scherer, M. J. (1993) *Living in the State of Stuck: How Assistive Technology Affects the Lives of People with Disabilities.* Brookline Books, Cambridge, MA; p. 189.

World Health Organization (1981) Health for All by the Year 2000: an alternative strategy. *World Health Forum* **2**: 500–511.

Evaluation in Community Based Rehabilitation

INTRODUCTION

There is a direct link between planning, management, programme operations and evaluation. An evaluation monitoring process for community based rehabilitation (CBR) programmes should be developed during the planning phase, before any activities are initiated. Evaluation is the process which will make it possible for the programme participants to measure the effectiveness of the CBR activities, and must be an integral and ongoing component of all programme activities.

Evaluation has been unfairly regarded as a negative or intimidating process associated with employment review, resource allocation and discontinuation of programme activities. Acceptance of evaluation as a component of the programme will help dispel the perception that evaluation is a threatening activity, that there is 'no time' to do it, or that appropriate skills are not available. It is important that all members of the CBR process are aware of the reasons for evaluation and the strategies to be employed and that their support and collaboration is vitally important (O'Toole *et al.*, 1995).

WHAT, HOW AND WHY TO EVALUATE

Even if management and planning of community rehabilitation services are based on the combined advice of local community leaders, professionals and planning experts, there is no assurance that the individual with a disability or the community will automatically benefit. The purpose of evaluation is to find out if the programme is accomplishing what it set out to do.

If the evaluation request comes from an outside source, the programme can organize the evaluation process so that the results are useful for programme planning. Whether the evaluation process is internally or externally motivated, ownership and involvement should come from the programme itself. Evaluation can be regarded as a systematic process of learning from the experiences of the programme and using this information to improve activities and promote effective planning by being able to select alternatives for the future.

The project management process must be quite clear:

♦ Why evaluate?
♦ For whom?
♦ What to evaluate?
♦ How to evaluate?

Why Evaluate?

The evaluation process will provide invaluable information on areas of activity as listed below.

♦ Assess whether the programme has had an impact on the target population.
♦ Determine the rate of progress and make adjustments to improve it.
♦ Provide the CBR participants with tools for measuring the effectiveness of their work.
♦ Assess the sustainability of the CBR project.
♦ Enable other workers in rehabilitation to learn from their experiences.
♦ Assess whether the programme is consistent with established policy and is influencing the development of related policy issues.
♦ Determine cost effectiveness.
♦ Determine whether a programme can be replicated or extended (Murthy et al., 1993).

For Whom?

All those involved in CBR have an interest in the evaluation process and its outcome. This includes:

♦ persons with disabilities;
♦ caregivers/family;

♦ community;
♦ employers;
♦ professional groups;
♦ government and policy agencies;
♦ donors;
♦ related health and social agencies (Helander, 1993).

What to Evaluate?

The design of the evaluation strategy is directly linked to the scope and variety of programme activities. As CBR varies significantly in its approach and complexity, the 'what to' evaluate will vary accordingly. The following are examples of what to evaluate:

♦ needs of the community and the target population;
♦ utilization of existing services, and quality of care;
♦ governance and management functions;
♦ financial and physical resources, cost effectiveness and cost benefits;
♦ human resources: staff selection, recruitment and training;
♦ relevance;
♦ impact, effectiveness and output (Murthy et al., 1993).

Needs of the community and the target population

The needs of the community will take into consideration the existing resources and the magnitude and variety of disability present. There are many methods which can be used to identify the disability needs of a community including surveys which report incidence and prevalence of disability, infrastructure and specific rehabilitation and vocational training requirements. In addition, informal inquiries with key informants can provide relevant background data.

The evaluation question of 'what percentage of the target population is covered by the CBR programme?' is

Table 7.1   Service components and quality of care indicators

Service components	Quality of care indicators
Acceptability	Consumer and professional satisfaction
Availability	Location and hours of service
Staff development	Training and internal mobility
Responsiveness	Information sharing and feedback to and from the community
Accessibility	Knowledge of services, appropriate referral, appropriate population, utilization
Comprehensiveness	Range of services and referral
Efficiency	Productivity and staff turnover
Services quality	Record keeping and continuity of care

answered by comparing the number of people identified as needing help to the number of people involved in the programme. If this kind of survey is carried out at the beginning of the programme, determining the extent of programme coverage is straightforward. Another way of estimating programme coverage is to use an available national statistic (3–7% of the target population being disabled is a standard statistic) and apply it to the population in an area.

Utilization of existing services, and quality of care
An evaluation should address a number of key service components and incorporate indicators of quality of care (Peat and Boyce, 1993) (Table 7.1)

Governance and management functions
The areas to be considered in governance and management functions include:

♦ strategic plan (statement of programme missions and goals);
♦ governance structures (committees and line of reporting);
♦ involvement of persons with disability;
♦ managerial training strategies;
♦ public relations;
♦ community networking.

Financial and physical resources – cost-effectiveness and cost benefits
The basis of financial evaluation of the CBR programme involves acquiring adequate and accurate financial information. The framework for data collection should be initiated at the onset, during the conception and planning phase of a programme. Some suggestions for the financial monitoring process are set out in Chapter 6. These include:

♦ standard budget accounting procedures;
♦ estimating and tracking community contributions;
♦ comparing community contributions to total operating costs;
♦ sources of funds for required continuing education and training;
♦ projections of financial needs over the next year/two years/three years.

Cost-effectiveness and cost benefit analyses compare costs or investments made in the CBR programme to the outcomes achieved. These calculations may require sophisticated financial analysis, however, elementary variations that are within the reach of CBR programmes include:

♦ *Cost per participant* is the total cost of the programme divided by the number of people who have used the service. This information is valuable when tracking the programme's cost effectiveness over time and when comparing one CBR programme to another.

♦ *Value of community contribution* is an estimation of the resources contributed to the CBR programme by the community. Donation of time, goods, services, materials, and money are included in this important figure. Equivalent costs of programme contributions are estimated by the amount that the programme would have paid if it went through commercial channels to receive the goods and services. For example, estimates are based on market value estimates of professional time, building materials, media coverage, food and volunteer work.

As stated in the previous chapter, the monitoring process for capturing this information should be established early on in the initial stages of programme implementation because it is this estimate that most tangibly demonstrates the community's motivation to sustain the project.

♦ *Cost and viability* are those costs that need to be covered by the local community which might include:
  – donations of support: for volunteers, such as training, transportation or seed money for income generating projects;
  – stationery and other office supplies for programme operations;
  – materials for assistive equipment such as ramps, mobility devices.

♦ *Programme costing* is an effective way to evaluate activities that the CBR programme wants to highlight. Activities are grouped along programme lines and may include:
  – community awareness activities;
  – monitoring and evaluation activities;
  – income generation activities;
  – training;
  – liaison with referral agencies, government departments;
  – management and communication activities.

Human resources – staff selection, recruitment, and training
Evaluation of activities includes the procedures used for staff selection and recruitment, induction and in-service training. It is important to identify whether job descriptions or task descriptions are adequately defined and available. All training programmes should be evaluated for both content and methods, from informal information sharing to prescribed educational programmes (Murthy *et al.*, 1993).

Relevance
Relevance refers to the meaning of CBR programme activities to the target group. A test of programme relevance determines whether CBR has addressed the needs of disabled people and their families and if its purpose remains valid and appropriate (Helander, 1993). Whether or not the programme collects data in order to conform to government guidelines may be irrelevant to the CBR community. What will have relevance is how the data related to community needs is collected, reviewed and shared with the community.

Impact and effectiveness and outcomes
Impact measures the wide scale effect of the programme on the community and various levels of government. Impact is usually discussed in terms of policies that enhance CBR activities and change attitudes toward disability. One measure of programme impact would be a determination of how the attitudes toward disability have changed. Intended as well as unintended outcomes are considered under this term. An unintended positive

outcome of the CBR disability prevention programme may be that the local elementary school in the region incorporates disability issues and prevention topics into the students' programme of studies.

Effectiveness means looking closely at the objectives that can be measured. An example of this would be a determination of the number of people with disabilities enrolled in the programme or the support received from professional groups. To determine the progress of the CBR programme, a comparison is made between activities that were planned and those carried out. Efficiency is made evident by comparing the programme results with resources expended.

How to Evaluate?

Systematic evaluation will only be adopted if there is a recognized need and if the methods are understood and applicable. The evaluation process includes the following:

- *Planning and preparation*: This includes the identification of the purpose of the evaluation, the approval of the process by the participants and an agreement on how to use the results. The plan should specify when evaluation is going to take place and by whom, and for how long.
- *Collection and monitoring of baseline data*: This term is frequently used to identify the collection of relevant and easily measurable information normally recorded in a quantitative manner, such as information on kind and number of programme activities, workers and attendance at events. Monitoring includes routine reporting, detailed activity plans and timetables and provides the basic framework for an evaluation. Baseline data can describe the situation before a programme starts and identify a point of reference from which progress can be measured.
- *Implementation*: There are five main mechanisms for obtaining the desired information:
  - collecting, tabulating, analysing already available data;
  - questioning through interviews;
  - conducting surveys;
  - direct observation of people and events;
  - analysis: evaluation is examining progress and changes and their significance in relationship to needs, existing services, impact, effectiveness, relevance, outcomes, and financial, human and physical resources.

QUANTITATIVE VERSUS QUALITATIVE DATA

Quantitative data can be precise but do not always reflect what was intended to be measured. These data include basic numeric information. The qualitative approach to data collection allows an evaluator to explore the meaning behind the people's perceptions and provides a systematic approach for gaining evidence from which insights can be drawn about persons with disabilities in the community. Qualitative data are useful in finding out how people think and feel, and their attitudes, beliefs and behaviours. These data are subjective in nature and in some instances may be biased, and therefore need to be balanced by objective, quantitative information.

USES OF EVALUATION FINDINGS

Planners, managers and community members must have access to evaluation data that they can trust and understand.

Evaluations are of little value if they are not used for decision-making purposes. There is wide evidence that evaluation recommendations should be:

♦ strong, plausible and suggest logical solutions;
♦ timely;
♦ a result of community involvement;
♦ clear and grounded in sound data;
♦ useful and practical.

Sustainability of a programme refers to whether there are adequate, appropriate and ongoing resources to continue programme activities. To be viable, the programme must have community support and acceptance. The ability of a programme to become sustainable depends to a large extent on how effectively it utilizes the findings of the ongoing evaluation process.

PARTICIPATORY EVALUATION

Recent experience has shown that evaluations are most useful when those who will make use of the results are involved in planning and implementation of the evaluation. Project managers, community members, programme participants, persons with disabilities and caregivers should have an active part in planning, implementing and using the results of an evaluation.

Participatory evaluation is a strategy which can reduce alienation and make evaluation more acceptable. It has the added benefit of involving people in the process who are familiar with the cultural, social and economic structure of the community. Wide representation and involvement in the process can be formalized through the formation of an Evaluation Steering Committee. At each critical juncture of the information collection and analysis, the Committee should be given feedback so that no surprises or alienation results at the end of the evaluation review (Jonsson, 1993). Figure 7.1 is a graphic representation of a sample work plan for participatory evaluation.

Participatory Rural Appraisal

Participatory rural appraisal (PRA) has been used in community development programmes in the areas of agriculture, income generation, literacy and community based rehabilitation. PRA is a technique which encourages community members to express and analyse information about their way of life and their local physical, social, economic and political environments to address disability issues. Although interviews, observation and questionnaires are the traditional methods of collecting data, PRA uses games and simulations to encourage the community to share their experiences and opinions about disability and community issues (Soeharso and Elip, 1995)

PRA in a CBR programme can assist in:

♦ identifying the priority disability issues and how these relate to community priorities;
♦ uncovering the community's knowledge and attitudes about disability; who is considered disabled; and what causes disability;
♦ identifying what services are available, and the degree to which these services are seen as effective and reliable (Soeharso and Elip, 1995).

MODELS OF EVALUATION

Models of evaluation abound, and although the terminology differs slightly, the basis and approach to comprehensive

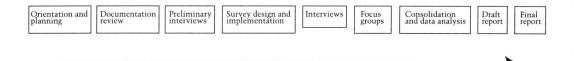

Figure 7.1   Community based rehabilitation: participatory evaluation work plan

Orientation and planning: Establish an Evaluation Steering Committee, and confirm the work plan.
Documentation review: Review documentation regarding programme goals and objectives, and determine aspects of the programme that can be evaluated.
Preliminary interviews: Conduct approximately 8 to 10 interviews with key informants, and select key questions.
Survey design and implementation: Develop questionnaire and letter of introduction, review questionnaire with staff, and distribute, collect and analyse data.
Interviews: Conduct approximately 30 interviews, consider what patterns emerge, determine expected use of findings.
Focus groups: Discuss key questions with important community members at five focus groups.
Consolidation and data analysis: Identify trends and issues.
Draft report: Prepare draft report and discuss with staff and key informants.
Final report: Review draft report, submit final report.
(Adapted from Department of Public Health, 1986).

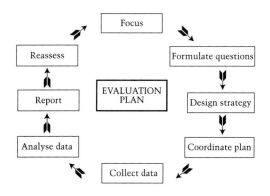

Figure 7.2   The eight stage model of evaluation (Department of Public Health, 1986).

evaluation remains remarkably constant. Figure 7.2 shows the evaluation review process.

According to the World Health Organization (WHO, 1981), 'Evaluation is a systematic way of learning from experience and using the lessons learned to improve current activities and promote better planning by a careful selection of alternatives for future action. This involves an analysis of different phases of a programme, its relevance, its formulation, its efficiency and effectiveness and its acceptance by all parties involved.'

REFERENCES

Department of Public Health, City of Toronto (1986) *The Evaluation Book: A Guide to Assessing Programs*: Toronto, Canada.

Helander, E. (1993) *Prejudice and Dignity: An Introduction to Community Based Rehabilitation*. United Nations Development Program, New York.

Jonsson, T. (1993) *Guide on Evaluation of Rehabilitation Programmes for Disabled People*. UNDP Interregional Program for Disabled People.

Murthy, R., Pruthvish, S. and Thomas, M. (1993) Evaluation of health programmes of non government organizations. Bangalore, India. *Action Aid Disability News* **4**(1): 16–19.

O'Toole, B., Krefting, L. and Gaudron, A. (1995). Unpublished paper *Guidelines for Evaluating Community Based Rehabilitation Programmes, Using Evaluation Information to Improve Programmes*.

Peat, M. and Boyce, W. (1993) Canadian community rehabilitation services: challenges for the future. *Canadian Journal of Rehabilitation* **6**(4): 281–289.

Soeharso, D. and Elip E. (1995) *Participatory Rural Appraisal*. Community based Reha-

bilitation Development and Training Centre, Solo, Central Java, Indonesia.

World Health Organization (1981) *Health Programme Evaluation, Guiding Principles*. WHO, Geneva.

Education in Community Based Rehabilitation

COMMUNITY BASED REHABILITATION KNOWLEDGE BASE

The development of community based rehabilitation (CBR) has produced a wide array of educational programmes and strategies extending from grassroots 'in service' one-on-one educational activities, to formal postgraduate education in the health science and university environment. For the most part, the knowledge and skill base of CBR has evolved from the experience of the non-government organization sector, as they have provided training programmes for the CBR worker, the volunteer and groups working at the community development level. In recent years, the education of health professionals and others working in the areas of disability and handicap has focused more on the clinical dimensions of community practice. The transfer of knowledge within the broad spectrum of CBR

should be viewed in the context of a continuum, extending from the person with a disability who may be acquiring new life skills, to the government policy-maker developing and implementing public policy related to disability and handicap.

'Rehabilitation includes all measures aimed at reducing the impact of disability for an individual enabling him or her to achieve independence, social integration, a better quality of life and self-actualization' (Helander, 1993). To accomplish such a broad objective requires a partnership between the various stakeholders in CBR. Effective communication among the stakeholders is therefore essential. In CBR, the education and training of a community volunteer are as important as the education of health professionals in community practice. Each has a unique role and occupies an important place in the spectrum of education and the transfer of knowledge and skills. It is therefore important that educators understand the different educational approaches that will be required if each of these stakeholders is to meet their objectives.

TRANSFER OF KNOWLEDGE AND SKILL

Many community practitioners are not aware of how much of the day-to-day work involves teaching. All community practitioners, whether volunteers, parents or health professionals, are teachers. Very often this role will be superimposed, or will run concurrently with other responsibilities. Community development activities have many approaches to teaching and employ a variety of learning strategies for the individual or for a gathering of people, in small and large group situations (Compton and Ashwin, 1993). Increasing knowledge also increases understanding. The transfer of knowledge provides a new framework of understanding which will enable persons with disability to perceive their situation differently and be able to manage themselves more appropriately. Education is a vital component of rehabilitation.

Many of the day-to-day aspects of CBR involve teaching. These can range from the explanation of the use of simple rehabilitation equipment to the development of comprehensive community education strategies to effect changes in attitudes toward disability. The educational needs of an individual or a community should be defined positively in terms of providing new opportunities and choices, and not by merely offering remedial and generic solutions to problems. Teachers need to be able to determine what they can contribute based on an assessment of their own personal and professional competencies, and the assessment of the capacities of the people with whom they interact and the situations in which training occurs. Effective education in CBR provides people with the skills and information to arrive at their own definition of rehabilitation and health, and to understand how to achieve these (Compton and Ashwin, 1993).

STAKEHOLDERS IN THE EDUCATIONAL PROCESS

The stakeholders in CBR are not only those who stand to benefit from the presence of CBR programmes, but are also all those involved in the design and delivery of the programme. The largest stakeholder in any educational programme is the community itself. The enhancement of the quality of life for persons with a disability, including their full integration into their communities and the provision of opportunities for employment, affects the family and society as a whole.

Persons with Disabilities
The person with a disability has a multidimensional role in education and is both recipient and participant in the CBR educational process. A vital component of the skill and knowledge base in CBR is the personal experience of the person with a disability. Any educational programme from the most simple to the most complex, must incorporate the collective experiences of persons with disabilities. The experience of the community of persons with a disability is a core element of the knowledge base and is a key factor in identifying the educational objectives and strategies of any educational or training programme. The development of public policies related to women with disabilities has been greatly advanced by the sharing of experiences of women in general, in terms of their struggle for equal opportunities in education and employment.

The person with a disability as a

teacher can be particularly effective in topic areas such as life skills. The personal and practical experience of a person with a disability in dealing with environmental issues, such as transportation and accessibility and social issues or the attitudes of employers, is part of the 'living laboratory' of CBR education.

Families/Caregivers

The family, as the primary caregivers, possess a distinctive knowledge base related to the nature of the essential daily support and personal needs of persons with disabilities. The family or caregivers, like the person with a disability, are both recipient of programmes, and participants in educational programmes that involve the transfer of knowledge and skills.

Community Members

The community, in both the geographic and social sense, is a critical stakeholder in the educational process. The experiences of a community in establishing programmes related to disability issues provide a record of successes and failures in community participation. The 'database' of community experience in a variety of social, cultural and economic situations should be integrated into the design of educational programmes in CBR. The experience of the community is relevant to understanding collective behaviour and to the design of education programmes.

Volunteers

One of the challenges of ongoing volunteer support is in providing the training and support which is critical for programme sustainability. As volunteers become more capable at disability identification and community education, they often realize a need for more comprehensive training that will permit them to deal more effectively with complex commu-

nity rehabilitation activities. Education alone does not ensure the success of volunteers or CBR programmes. However, education advances the development of interpersonal skills, basic literacy, general knowledge and practical skills. The most important aspect of voluntarism is the personal characteristics of volunteers – their patience, commitment and communication skills. One of the strongest motivators for volunteering is the increased knowledge and skills that the volunteer acquires through CBR training programmes (Lysack, 1992).

CBR Workers/CBR Supervisors

The CBR workers, excluding persons with disabilities and their families, are the primary personnel in grassroots programmes and provide CBR education and training and other support services. The CBR worker in the role of teacher or trainer is a principal stakeholder in the educational process. The CBR worker interacts at a variety of levels from a one-to-one educational activity to providing group training programmes.

Government and Multilateral Agencies

Educational strategies in government and multilateral sectors have included disability prevention programmes such as the WHO and national government initiatives focusing on the eradication of poliomyelitis and increasing public awareness of the major preventable causes of disabilities. The recent emphasis placed on the development of CBR in post-conflict situations by the World Bank illustrates the need for multilateral agencies to develop rehabilitation programmes at the community level which will deal effectively with the disability crises created in areas of conflict. The development of public policy related to disability issues is a result of the educational partnership between community stakeholders, including persons with disabilities, the community, non-government and multilateral agencies and government policy-makers. These agencies are therefore stakeholders in the educational process as recipients of information, providers of public educational programmes and facilitators in the development of public policy.

Health Care and Related Professionals

Traditional professional education programmes have produced clinicians for institutional practice settings. Now that health and social policy-makers and planners, and international non-government agencies seem to be agreeing that more services should be provided in community settings, the concept of community based professional training and education is an important trend in current methods of education. To be most effective, the philosophy of CBR and health care must be integrated into the learning process of health care professionals so that in their practice they are responsive to the rehabilitation and health care needs and societal values of the communities they serve.

The majority of professionals would still view the traditional institutional setting as their preferred option for practice. However, universities and other educational institutions are now more sensitive to their 'community' role and are designing educational experiences for practitioners which incorporate community priorities and development issues. The institutions providing professional education perceive themselves as major stakeholders in producing future professionals, and providing educational programmes to meet community rehabilitation needs.

Recently Canadian professional educational institutions have become more involved in the provision of educational programmes for non-professionals such as personnel from non-government organization CBR programmes. Professional institutions are beginning to see themselves as major stakeholders in the provision of education and training for non-professional groups and the development of learning resources for personnel at the community level.

Employers

Public policy, public education programmes and vocational training initiatives have made the private sector more aware that people with a disability are a viable and integral part of the social and economic environment. Traditionally, however, persons with disabilities have been 'the last to be hired and the first to be fired' (Disabled People's International, 1993). Therefore, educational programmes must target the employment sector in order to increase its understanding and perceptions of the viability of employing persons with a disability and integrating them into the economic life of the community.

STRATEGIES IN EDUCATION

There are a number of educational options and strategies in CBR just as there are many different approaches to the implementation of CBR. These include:

- The acquisition of knowledge and skills through work in the community with no formal educational process;
- Structured courses for CBR workers lasting a few days;
- Programmes for CBR workers of several weeks' or months' duration;
- Programmes for CBR workers of a year or more;
- Professional education in CBR at the undergraduate level;
- Professional education in CBR at the postgraduate level;

- Advanced education in CBR for policy-makers and managers.

Similarly, when classifying CBR workers, there is again a broad range of levels of involvement and categories of employment. The major areas include:

- CBR volunteer worker on a casual basis;
- CBR worker with daily responsibilities;
- CBR trainer who provides instruction for the first level worker, but who may also function as a CBR worker with daily responsibilities;
- CBR trainer of trainers, whose primary function is the provision of educational programmes for CBR workers;
- CBR manager and administrator;
- health and other professionals with a major commitment to CBR;
- government personnel responsible for policy development and implementation in CBR.

As there is no single approach that can be recognized as 'CBR education,' and no single strategy for educating any one level of CBR worker, it is important that the design of educational programmes be driven by the needs of the community, the background and experiences of the participants, the unique objectives of the programme, and the human and financial resources available. Education strategies can include a combination of approach and techniques.

Approach
- One-on-one demonstration
- Seminars
- Didactic teaching
- Discussion groups
- Practicum

Techniques
- Independent learning

- Ongoing/lifelong learning
- Problem solving
- Continuing education

CRITICAL FACTORS IN THE DESIGN AND IMPLEMENTATION OF CBR EDUCATIONAL PROGRAMMES

The following is based on the recommendations developed by a symposium in training courses in CBR conducted in Uppsala, Sweden in 1995. These recommendations review the major factors to be taken into consideration when planning a course, designing curricula, and choosing educational strategies in CBR.

General Criteria for Site Selection

The criteria for selection of a training site for CBR educational programmes include:

- well-functioning CBR programme in government and non-government sectors;
- community development programmes related to disability and handicap;
- active participation of people with disabilities;
- possible collaboration with other educational programmes or facilities.

Planning of Courses

Before a training course is initiated it is important to determine:

- the participants' background;
- the type of training to be given (community development, rehabilitation/ therapeutic skills, management or combination of these);

◆ where the course is to be performed (national, regional, or international).

Core Curriculum Issues

In all training programmes it is important to consider the knowledge, skills and attitudes of participants. Specific topics to be included in training programmes for CBR coordinators or managers are:

◆ CBR concepts and practices, including planning, implementation, monitoring and evaluation, clear multi-sector content;
◆ the relationship between CBR and community development;
◆ attitudes about disability issues and disabled people's organizations;
◆ community participation;
◆ networking and coordination;
◆ implementation of the 'UNDP Standard Rules';[1]
◆ social marketing and community education;
◆ interpersonal and communication skills;
◆ training and methodology;
◆ financial management and personnel management;
◆ supervision and consultancy;
◆ advocacy.

Organization of Training

The criterion for the selection of participants depends upon the level of the course. Selection of participants for enrolment in national and international courses should consider the following:

◆ the sector from which the participants come (non-government organizations, governmental sector or health and education);
◆ experience of community development and/or experience in work with disabled people;
◆ whether there is active recruitment of people with disabilities.

Courses for the constituents
There should be a set of courses available for different sectors (senior civil servants, programme managers, professionals). The interdependence of community level workers and different professionals should be made clear and demonstrated.

Link to universities/colleges and international programmes
Universities and colleges in developed and developing countries should actively promote CBR (or community disability services) in their own countries. International courses should encourage research and training. International research training courses should include a review of issues related to research ethics (Uppsala Conference, 1995).

POTENTIAL PROBLEMS IN CBR TRAINING PROGRAMMES

The workshop on CBR held in Bangalore, India 1992 (Seva-in-Action), identified the following as important issues related to design and location of training programmes:

◆ *Centralized training*: a centralized training programme with facilities

---

[1] Refers to the Standard Rules in United Nations Development Program (1991), Division for Global and Interregional Programs, *Disabled People's Participation in Sustainable Human Development*.

and resources and a developed infrastructure can provide a comprehensive approach to education. However, centralized programmes would seem to work 'at odds' with the CBR philosophy, as they are often inaccessible geographically and economically to a large number of CBR personnel. Decentralized programmes such as 'itinerant teaching teams' could be more effective in terms of providing training to many people in an accessible way. However, the lack of an infrastructure in the decentralized approach could adversely affect the quality of the programme.

♦ *Training people to be trainers*: many of those proficient in various areas of rehabilitation do not possess the necessary skills to transfer their knowledge to others. The ability to transfer skill is in itself a skill and therefore should be taken into consideration in the design and implementation of training programmes.

EDUCATIONAL SYSTEMS IN CBR

Education through Experience

The acquisition of knowledge and skills related to disability and handicap occurs not only through organized educational programmes, but through day-to-day personal experience and the development of life skills. Therefore, those who are participants in, or observers of, the wide range of CBR activities increase their knowledge and skill through personal involvement. Family members of disabled persons and caregivers acquire a great deal of their skill and understanding through meeting the daily needs of the person with a disability. In fact, in many instances, family members may be the most knowledgeable group in identifying

the strategies which are most appropriate and effective in the development of community rehabilitation services and educational programmes. Many non-government organizations provide outstanding CBR programmes and have developed innovative, cost-effective, and sustainable projects without access to any formal educational resource. The real life experiences and acquired knowledge of the person with a disability and their caregivers have been their major resource.

Non-professional Education and Training

A wide variety of terms are used in describing the different roles and responsibilities of the human resource base of CBR. The following identifies the broad general categories of community personnel:

♦ Community worker
♦ Community supervisor
♦ Trainer of trainers

Training for Community Workers

A key role in the CBR approach is played by the community workers, also referred to as 'village health worker' or 'local supervisor'. The success of a CBR programme rests on the quality of training of locally recruited, first-level supervisors who serve as non-professional case managers. Community workers can receive comprehensive information related to the vocational, educational, medical, and social needs of persons with disabilities, as well as more specialized knowledge and skills (Helander *et al.*, 1989). The extent of the responsibilities of a community worker is decided by the community, and the extent of the responsibilities assigned depends on factors such as what personnel and services are already available in the community and what needs and objectives are identified by the community. Most programmes focus on one constituency (elderly, children) and/or on a particular clinical issue (orthopaedics or poliomyelitis) (Pickles, 1989). The learning and teaching processes are central to community based programmes where the person with a disability or those providing care for the person with a disability, learn basic procedures and how to adapt to living with a disability in order to achieve as much functional independence as possible. Broader community education undertaken by community supervisors aims to remove or reduce societal barriers to independence, and increase awareness of health promotion and disability prevention.

The United Nations Development Programme, as part of their programme for the Decade of Disabled Persons, sponsored the development of a manual for *Training in the Community for People with Disabilities* (Helander *et al.*, 1989). This document was prepared for people in the community who were planning, implementing or evaluating CBR programmes and consists of 34 modules and 30 training packages for community workers who implement programmes, community rehabilitation committee members who help manage programmes, and others such as school teachers who assist children with disabilities. The manual has four guides, one of which is written for persons with disabilities, describing what they can do for themselves and for others in the community. The packages deal with different disability topics (visual impairment, hearing loss, learning difficulties etc.) and provide basic information on activities of daily living and rehabilitation procedures, as well as social and vocational activities. When translated into local dialects, this manual has been an invaluable resource

for all stakeholders in the CBR process, but of greatest value to the community worker.

Although there are many models for the training of community workers, the example shown in Figure 8.1 proposes a modular approach to a ten-week course, which could be adjusted to suit local conditions and needs. Community workers who would take this course are most likely to have been recruited by their own community, employed or compensated by it, and receive their managerial supervision from a local committee.

Training a worker who comes from the community, ensures that the service provided to the community will be by an individual who understands the cultural biases of a person with a disability. The following programmes are designed to provide local supervisors, or community workers recruited from the community with training, so they in turn will train family members to assist a disabled relative appropriately.

Training curriculum and training module for CBR personnel, Bangalore, India (Action Aid)

It was proposed that a curriculum and training model be developed to bring some uniformity in the pattern of training for CBR workers. Sourabha, the CBR project of Sri Ramana Maharishi Academy for the Blind, and Action Aid, jointly designed an educational programme for community workers. The objectives of this programme are to enable the CBR worker to achieve a minimum level of competency in the following areas:

- cerebral palsy;
- locomotor disabilities;
- communication disabilities;
- visual impairment.

Example of Training Programme for Local Community Supervisors

WEEK   COURSE CONTENT
One:
   ♦ Course evaluation and requirements to pass.
   ♦ Perceptions and definitions of disabled people.
   ♦ General interventions: functional training, education, vocational training, jobs, protection of human rights, organizing people, social integration. Role of community initiatives.
   ♦ Community organizations for development.

Two:
   ♦ Local survey (theory and practice).
   ♦ Assessment of disabled people.

Three:
   ♦ Seeing difficulties. Meet blind people, practice, schooling, jobs.
   ♦ Referrals.

Four:
   ♦ Hearing and speech difficulties. Meet deaf/mute people, practice, schooling, jobs.
   ♦ Referrals.

Five:
   ♦ Moving difficulties. Meet persons with disabilities, practice, including prevention of deformities.

Six:
   ♦ Make walking aids and other technical appliances.

Seven:
   ♦ Schooling, jobs.
   ♦ Referrals.

Eight:
   ♦ Feeling difficulties (leprosy); strange behaviour (mental disease); learning difficulties (mental retardation), practice, schooling, jobs.
   ♦ Referrals.

Nine:
   ♦ Child development; play activities; multihandicapped; role of local healers.

Ten:
   ♦ Education of children with special needs; adult education.
   ♦ Social activities, household activities.
   ♦ Income generation and market situation.
   ♦ Simple assessment.
   ♦ Informal vocational training.
   ♦ Employment and self-employment opportunities.
   ♦ Protection of human rights.
   ♦ Organizations of disabled persons.
   ♦ Reporting, recording, filing, and in-service training.

(Adapted from Helander, 1993).

Figure 8.1

The curriculum focuses on issues such as:

♦ identification;
♦ assessment;
♦ referral;
♦ follow-up;
♦ therapy;
♦ education;
♦ vocational training; and
♦ placement.

The programme was organized on the basis of one day per week session (Pruthvish and Rajendra, 1993):

10 sessions	Mental retardation, cerebral palsy and muscular dystrophy
10 sessions	Speech and hearing disabilities
6 sessions	Locomotor disabilities
8 sessions	Visual disabilities
4 sessions	Management of CBR programmes

Introductory training for CBR and community development, CBR Development and Training Centre, Colomdu, Solo, Indonesia
This is a programme for people with community development experience in assisting persons with disabilities. The course lasts 12 weeks and is conducted in English with a course limit of 10–15 participants.

Training for 'Teachers of Teachers', Managers and Coordinators
Managers, coordinators and trainers of trainers programmes will require more comprehensive curricula than those available for a general introduction to CBR and for the training of community workers. An example of this type of programme is the one offered at the Institute of Child Health, London. This institution offers a nine-month diploma course and is targeted at trainers and managers of CBR programmes in developing countries.
The curriculum includes:

♦ basic health skills in the rehabilitation sciences;
♦ prevention of disability;
♦ diagnosis and evaluation of disability;
♦ epidemiology and statistics;
♦ management skills;
♦ practical sociology;
♦ growth and development;
♦ education of the disabled child;
♦ mobility, simple aids and equipment;
♦ detection and measurement of visual or hearing defects; and
♦ economics of rehabilitation.

A review of other courses illustrates the type of topic which can be included in this level of programme:

♦ self-advocacy;
♦ design and production of low cost aids;
♦ vocational rehabilitation;
♦ income generation;
♦ developmental education;
♦ distance education strategies;
♦ social marketing;
♦ social change and critical awareness;
♦ multicultural education.

In *Community Care for Health Professionals*, Compton and Ashwin (1994) refer to the 'ten commandments for community teachers' (Figure 8.2). These guidelines for the teachers of community teachers can also be applied to the education of community workers by professionals, and to the education of the person with a disability, their family and the community by the health care worker.

Professional Education Programmes

Curriculum content in undergraduate education programmes provides a sound

Ten Commandments for Community Teachers.

1   Teaching must be a response to clearly identified needs.
2   What is taught must be seen to have relevance to the life of the learner.
3   Learners must be engaged and involved in the learning experience.
4   The goals of each learning session must be identified and made known to the learner.
5   The goals should be sufficient without being overwhelming.
6   The language should be clear and have meaning for the learner.
7   Teaching begins with what is familiar before moving to what is unfamiliar.
8   There should be variety in presentation to maintain interest and increase retention.
9   Learning should be clearly structured to aid assimilation.
10 Ways of evaluating outcomes should be devised before the teaching programme begins.

Figure 8.2

knowledge base in educating rehabilitation professionals. These programmes focus on basic science and clinical practice issues. It is recognized that in addition to preparing the practitioner for the clinical role, educational programmes will need to develop or enhance the undergraduate curriculum in the areas of communication, teaching, networking, counselling, advocacy, health promotion and administrative and management skills. An important feature of education will be increasing health care professionals, awareness of cultural differences, attitudes, beliefs and behaviours with regard to disablement and persons with disabilities (Pickles, 1989). Rehabilitation therapy is no longer limited to traditional institutional practice. Future professionals must be educated to assume leadership roles in community practice settings alongside various community agencies, services and other professionals, in ways that are culturally and socially appropriate.

A number of university programmes educating rehabilitation professionals, now include specific curriculum components dealing with community based practice. For example, in Ontario, Canada, in order to meet the requirements for accreditation and thus the continuation of undergraduate programmes, curricula must show that they are preparing physical therapists for practice in community settings (Canadian Directors of Physiotherapy Academic Programs, 1995). Queen's University includes a one-semester (12 weeks, for three hours per week) course dealing specifically with community practice. This course examines current models of community practice and focuses on the knowledge needed to provide occupational therapy and physical therapy in a community setting.

Topics discussed in this undergraduate CBR course include:

♦   models of community practice;
♦   community living, needs, coping, quality of life;
♦   considering culture in community practice;
♦   socioeconomic, literacy and lifestyle issues;
♦   health and disability;
♦   advocacy and human rights;
♦   consulting and networking;
♦   community roles for health professionals in non-traditional settings;
♦   social marketing (sharing health messages);
♦   health promotion – principles and applications;

♦ in addition to the formal didactic lectures, new and innovative community clinical placement opportunities are being provided as part of the education of rehabilitation therapy students.

The Pramukhswami Medical College, Kramsad, Gujarat, India is a rurally located medical college that was instituted in 1987 with the objective of preparing 'social doctors' proficient in rural, community based health care delivery with an emphasis on preventive and promotive health care. Conventional hospital based learning is supplemented and reinforced by intensive community based teaching and learning (Bansal *et al.*, 1994). The community based education of medical students starts from the entry into college. The overall programme includes:

♦ first year students visit villages once a week to participate in voluntary agency programmes;
♦ family health care, which provides students with the opportunity to study, analyse and provide health care to families in real life situations in communities;
♦ epidemiological visits, during third year to study a case of public importance;
♦ community posting programme in the final year of study, where students are posted for 30 days to study health problems of rural people and factors bearing on health status at the Department of Community Medicine.

Seth G. S. Medical College, University of Bombay, India, also provides community clinical education opportunities for occupational therapy and physical therapy students. This programme provides senior year students with practical experience in CBR programmes in both rural and urban environments. Students are provided with an opportunity of working within the framework of both institutional outreach programmes and CBR initiatives organized by local non-government organizations. The objective of the programme is to enhance the understanding and appreciation of community practice as a viable area of professional involvement.

The School of Physiotherapy and Occupational Therapy, University of Sri Lanka, has implemented a community field training programme. The programme for educating physiotherapists and occupational therapists in Sri Lanka and the rehabilitation service delivery model are patterned after the Western medical model. The School of Physiotherapy and Occupational Therapy felt therapists should be introduced into patients' homes while the students were still in training. This would serve the dual purpose of preparing them for future changes, as well as make their education more complete. A three-month training programme was introduced into the curriculum with the following objectives:

♦ to give students experience in the concept of total patient care;
♦ to familiarize students with the problems faced by persons with disabilities in the community, particularly in the activities of daily living;
♦ to prepare students to practise the specialties for which they are being trained in the environment of the patient's own home;
♦ to prepare students to detect physical disability in the community;
♦ to enable students to work with a health team in the community;
♦ to make students aware of community health problems (Fernando and Mendis, 1980).

Continuing Education and Distance Learning

Continuing education in CBR strategies for health professionals is necessary in order to expand and enhance the professional role in CBR. The Southampton Institute of Higher Education, Southampton, UK, Community Physiotherapy, designed a part-time course which was made available to experienced physiotherapists who had completed an introductory level course in CBR. The course provides clinicians with the opportunity to develop further the knowledge and skills required for successful performance as community physiotherapists in the United Kingdom. The course was developed by Southampton in cooperation with the Association of Community Chartered Physiotherapists and requires ten days of study, and five days of full-time placement with an experienced community physiotherapist who acts as a consultant.

The course objectives are:

♦ to provide an overview of CBR;
♦ to develop and encourage the necessary attitudes for efficient multidisciplinary care;
♦ to introduce the relevant knowledge and skills required to enable physiotherapists to work effectively and competently in the community (Pickles, 1989).

A programme conducted as 'distance learning' is being offered by the Centre for Educational Needs, Oxford Road, University of Manchester, England. The course is a 12-week programme available to those holding a qualification from a recognized university who have experience working with persons with disabilities and who are professionals in fields such as physical therapy, occupational therapy, nursing and social work.

Advanced and Interdisciplinary Graduate Level Education for Planners, Researchers, Policy Developers and Educators of Professionals

Educational programmes of this type explore philosophies and practices of rehabilitation, and non-traditional models of rehabilitation service delivery and manpower utilization. Study programmes involve a review of factors that affect and influence the rehabilitation process such as culture, ethical considerations and economics. Programmes with the greatest potential are those that do not limit entry to rehabilitation therapy professionals only, and that are developed to attract professionals and scientists in rehabilitation related disciplines who wish to pursue an interdisciplinary programme of study. This integrated approach to advanced education will have the added benefit of producing future rehabilitation personnel who will have a diverse and comprehensive view of the development of CBR (Pickles, 1989).

The School of Rehabilitation Therapy, Queen's University, Kingston, Ontario, Canada, offers a multidisciplinary Master of Science programme in Rehabilitation in which the student can focus on education and research related to CBR. This research-oriented degree programme is normally completed in two years and includes course work and the production of a research thesis. The programme is open to a variety of rehabilitation related disciplines including, but not limited to, occupational therapists, physical therapists, psychologists, sociologists, biomedical engineers and physicians.

The programme seeks to:

♦ provide the knowledge base and skills to develop a research project in community based rehabilitation;

- encourage a multidisciplinary approach to research;
- add to the scientific knowledge base in community based rehabilitation.

The Centre for Adult and Higher Education, University of Manchester, England provides a graduate Master of Education programme for those who will be, or are already, responsible for the educational dimension of primary health care programmes in developing countries. The education of professionals and the promotion of a learning process in the community are the two main elements of the course.

Course components include:

- Primary health care as education for development;
- Community health education;
- Management and planning of primary health care;
- Community based rehabilitation is available as a programme option.

In addition, the Institute of Child Health, University of London, offers a Master of Science programme with a specialization in Community Disability Studies. This is a one-year degree programme which accepts candidates with a combination of academic and appropriate experience background.

In summary, CBR initiatives, governments and other agencies are expressing the need for trained manpower. This has led to the development of educational programmes at a variety of levels. One of the essential elements of CBR is effective training and education of community workers, managers or coordinators of programmes, committee members, community members, persons with disabilities and their families. In addition, the future development of CBR will be strongly influenced by the rehabilitation scientist who advances the knowledge base in the rehabilitation disciplines, and who assumes leadership roles in public policy-making and planning for the future of rehabilitation.

REFERENCES

Arsenault, F. (1995) *From Clients to Consumers: The Canadian Disability Rights Movement*, Atlanta Conference Paper, International Centre for the Advancement of Community Based Rehabilitation, Queen's University, Canada.

Bansal, R. K., Arya, P. K., Sharma V. and Srivastava R. K. (1994) Community-based medical education: A case study of Pramukhswami Medical College. *NU News of Health Care in Developing Countries*. Vol. 8.

Canadian Directors of Physiotherapy Academic Programs (CDPAP) (1995). Curriculum for University Physiotherapy Programs, Canada.

Compton, A. and Ashwin, M. (1993) Community care for health professionals. In *Teaching in the Community*. Butterworth-Heinemann, London.

Disabled People's International (1993) Promotional brochure on DPI. DPI, Winnipeg, Manitoba, Canada.

Fernando, T. and Mendis, P. (1980) A community field training programme for students of physiotherapy and occupational therapy in Sri Lanka. *Physiotherapy* 66: 14.

Gloag, D. (1992) Severe disability: residential care and living in the community. *British Medical Journal* 290: 368–371.

Helander, E. (1993) *Prejudice and Dignity: An Introduction to Community Based Rehabilitation*. United Nations Development Program, New York.

Helander, E., Mendis, P., Nelson, G. and Goerdt, A. (1989) *Training in the Community for People with Disabilities*. WHO, Geneva.

Lysack, C. (1992) Community-based rehabilitation and volunteerism: an Indonesian experience with the motivation of volunteer workers. Master's Thesis, Queen's University, Canada.

NORAD, Seva-in-Action (1992) Community Based Rehabilitation Workshop. *Sharing Strengths*. Bangalore, India.

Pickles, B. (1989) Education for community based rehabilitation. In *Community Based Rehabilitation: International Perspectives* (monograph). Queen's University, Canada.

Pruthvish, S. and Rajendra K. K. (1993) *Development of a Training Curriculum and Training Module for CBR Personnel. Outlines of Proposed Methodology*. Sourabha and Action Aid, Bangalore, India.

Uppsala Conference (1995) *Symposium on Training Courses in Community Based Rehabilitation* June 12–16, Reprocentralen HSC, University of Uppsala, Sweden.

chapter
nine

The Economic and Social Consequences of Disability, and the Organization of Persons with Disabilities

INTRODUCTION

Too often in the past, health care policies and systems have been developed and implemented without an appreciation and understanding of the needs and complexities of the societies they serve. In community based rehabilitation (CBR) an essential feature is the full involvement of persons with disabilities in all aspects of programme design, implementation and evaluation. Within this framework it is essential to review the needs and aspirations of disabled persons and the history of the development of the consumer movement. It is not a new phenomenon to have persons with disabil-

ities within societies (Arsenault, 1993). What is a new phenomenon, however, is that persons with disabilities are now representing themselves to decision-makers at national and international levels, advocating the adoption of public policies which will enhance the inclusion of persons with disabilities, their families and communities.

Most of the common practices of society have a 'non-disabled' bias, and the social norms used to interpret and describe events and perceptions are based on the experiences of non-disabled persons. This is due in part to the fact that many of society's values and customs have been developed without any consideration for the participation of persons with disabilities in all systems which make up society (Arsenault, 1993). While this exclusion in some instances is not intentional, it has worked to marginalize persons with disabilities and prevent them from enjoying equal opportunities in the areas of education, employment and recreation. The exclusion of persons with disability has therefore affected the quality of their lives and the lives of their caregivers and families. Frequently, individuals who are disabled live in poverty because of the physical inaccessibility of the workplace and are also affected by stigmatization and negative attitudes.

By organizing themselves, people with disabilities have been able to articulate their views on issues related to handicap and disability. In the consumer movement, people with disabilities share their experiences and this sharing of individual personal histories has raised the awareness of society to the needs and aspirations of persons with disabilities. Arsenault in 1993 stated that:

As you hear more and more people explain that they have problems similar to ones you have, you realize that inaccessibility and exclusion are not your personal problems. Once this happens, it is not too long before people are strategizing about how they can change this situation to make improvements for themselves and others like them.

In a number of countries in the 1960s and 1970s, persons with disabilities discovered that they shared many common problems and decided to do something about it. What followed was the development of organizations representative of disability groups and issues. Collectively they could apply the pressure needed to attain full and equal participation for persons with disabilities. Disabled persons learned that they too had rights – the same rights as all other citizens (COPOH,

1991). In Canada, the establishment of the Coalition of Provincial Organizations of the Handicapped (COPOH) in 1976 was an excellent example of this successful organizational development.

In 1981, Henry H. Enns stated the position of disabled persons quite simply and directly when he said, 'They wanted to have the opportunity for full and equal participation in society' (Arsenault, 1993). To make that possible, attitudinal and architectural barriers would have to be eliminated. Disabled persons talked as citizens with rights and not as clients in need of services. In order to change the stereotype, persons with disabilities needed to change their own perception of their abilities and disabilities before they could begin to change the attitudes and beliefs of others. Some action-oriented individuals realized that the solution to many problems could be found within the strengths and resources of the community of persons with disabilities and organizations who could advocate for equal rights and opportunities.

Persons with disabilities felt that the existing service model viewed them as 'obedient and dependent' patients but not necessarily 'productive and independent' members of the community. Persons with disabilities wanted to make decisions about their own lives, the services they want, products they need, and changes they want to be made. They realized that only through their own direct involvement would the environment be made more accessible and safer for themselves.

ECONOMICS OF DISABILITY

Persons with a disability possess the talents, skills and capabilities to be active in a community and competitive in the workforce. They have a political force as voters, advocates and lobbyists active in social, economic and political life and are a market force as consumers of goods and services. They are also a labour force as employees and employers – particularly so in those societies increasingly conducive to their full participation.

Persons with a disability are frequently an untapped economic and social resource. Billions of dollars in social support are targeted annually for programmes aimed at serving the needs of persons with disabilities, their families and caregivers. However, a significant proportion of available financial resources are directed at health and social programmes which foster dependency. Although significant advances have been made recently to promote independence and empowerment, persons with disabilities are still the last into the workforce and the first to leave (Edmonds and Peat, 1996).

Costs of Disability

Costs to the System

One of the largest problems facing all societies today is the rapidly escalating cost of health care. While a lack of funds was more conventionally associated with health problems of less developed societies, the high cost of highly specialized care in more developed countries has become a great concern. Although governments have now taken a zero tolerance stand on hospital deficit financing, a complex and expensive infrastructure is still being maintained. Hospitals in many countries are funded on a global basis which involves allocating resources based on past utilization. Funding flows to where the providers, rather than the patients, are located. Many demands are being placed on the delivery of rehabilitation services and more and more

resources are being allocated to increasingly sophisticated techniques that are carried out in institutions. This only serves to increase the public's demand for costly services that often are available to only a small percentage of the population. The emphasis which has been placed on institutional care must be re-examined in the context of the requirements of the entire population and the most appropriate use of public health funds.

The development of health systems that concentrate on high technologies has hindered the development and implementation of services that can serve the broader population of persons with disabilities in the communities where they live. Rehabilitation technology in institutional settings is expensive and sophisticated and is only required by a few. In both less and more developed countries, the majority of the population in need of rehabilitation do not require sophisticated technology. In less developed countries, disabilities are largely the result of preventable diseases, while in more developed countries, disability is most often associated with ageing. In both less and more developed countries, services are often inaccessible. Figures 9.1 and 9.2 show that the majority of people with disabilities worldwide live in rural areas (Peat and Boyce, 1993).

Financial management of rehabilitation programmes is a concern for the policy-makers and budget-advisers who are responsible for operating rehabilitation programmes in a financially responsible and organized manner. Escalating costs of specialized services within a complex and expensive infrastructure are making it imperative for institutions and professionals to explore new approaches to the organization and delivery of rehabilitation and social services and to utilize the human resource base more effectively (Edmonds and Peat, 1996). The dichotomy

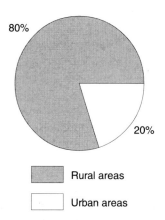

Figure 9.1 World's disabled in rural areas (Helander, 1993).

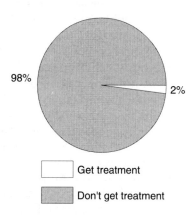

Figure 9.2 Persons with disabilities in rural areas (only 2% obtain treatment) (Helander, 1993).

of the present situation is the need to 'downsize' health and social systems on one hand and to maintain, or in fact increase, accessibility and quality on the other.

Loss of Skill and Experience

Though the costs of special education programmes for children with disabilities are twice the costs of the education for non-disabled children, the contribution of the rehabilitated and employed person is many times the cost of special education. The costs of special education are minimal when compared to the costs of institutionalization. (UNESCO, 1978)

Disability can have serious financial implications for industry in terms of labour turnover and the retraining of new workers. The volume of this loss is greater in developed countries where a much higher percentage of disabled persons will have received training and skills prior to disablement. In many instances, the disabled person within the labour force has less flexibility than other workers and so is more at risk of losing job skills when a change in employment situation occurs, when labour market conditions are altered or when new technologies are introduced. Disability also produces a secondary effect, as it is likely to affect the employment of caregivers and family members close to the disabled person. Productivity may also be affected by secondary emotional disturbance, stress and other psychosocial issues that lead to a decreased work output.

The implications of disability also depend on the unique political characteristics of a country, such as labour legislation, social security and subsidized or sheltered employment. The cost of disability will be greatest where nations are increasing the numbers in the active workforce. Unfortunately, the experience in some industrial countries is that older workers and the disabled are paid costly pensions to encourage them to leave the labour market to create places for new workers. There are significant social costs in this situation (Hammerman and Maikowski, 1981).

Measuring the Implications

The effects of disability on the workforce and income distribution can be measured using the following data in an analysis:

♦ absolute number of disabled;

- incidence of disability in different age groups;
- the type and degree of handicap;
- percentage of disabled who leave the workforce;
- labour force participation rate of disabled versus non-disabled;
- employment rate of adults in households with a disabled family member versus that of adults in households without such a member;
- household income data comparing households with, and those without a person with a disability;
- percentage of disabled who never enter the workforce;
- prevalence and incidence of disability.

The philosophy of CBR is to support the continuation of the person with a disability in the workforce as a viable and fully contributing member of society. CBR strategies must include programmes which facilitate the re-entry of persons with a disability into the workforce. Those with the most success are consistent with the International Labour Organization polices and the concepts of community based vocational training.[1]

Planners and policy-makers are challenged to identify and implement approaches which effectively utilize finite financial resources, and which will provide a foundation for health reform, improved health status and quality of life for persons with disabilities. CBR aims to influence the opportunity for persons with disability to live and work in their chosen environment and field of activity.

Costs to the Individual with a Disability

. . . those of us with disabilities struggle daily to be a part of our communities. We often live with poverty . . . we live with inadequate support systems that often leave us no alternative but to be housed in an institution. We live with an unemployment rate of 80% and we live in a society that continues to offer us pity and charity, not equality. (Arsenault, 1993)

Many activities of daily living that are available and financially accessible to most members of society are costly to those who have some form of disability. For example, transportation alternatives, communication aids, recreational availability, access to education, vocational options and choices in self-care assistance are just some of the many costly issues with which persons with a disability must deal. The costs to the individual with a disability often perpetuate dependency. Adults with a disability in all countries have difficulty obtaining appropriate training and education, finding jobs that pay adequately and accessing the employment environment. Children with disabilities seldom enjoy the same educational opportunities as other children. In a situation of poverty children with disabilities are more likely to become malnourished, are often weaker and have higher mortality rates.

Costs to the Family

In most communities, the family is a basic social unit in which each member has specific roles and responsibilities. The disablement of one member affects the whole family. It is suggested that families with a disabled member have greater financial stress, more frequent disruption of family routine and leisure, and poorer social interaction. In all societies, families carry the responsibility for their

---

[1] In Chapter 4, community based vocational rehabilitation and the International Labour Organization are reviewed in greater detail.

disabled members, which is costly to them financially, physically and emotionally. The actual cost of a disability is dependent on the cultural context. Attitudes and behaviours towards disability can affect the cost of a disability to the family and to society. When considering the family members of a disabled person, the conclusions of a United Nations report confirmed that a disability affects 25% of the world's population (UN Expert Meeting, 1977), as a person with a disability is to some extent dependent upon others. The whole life situation of persons with disabilities is shaped by how the immediate caregivers are able to cope with the problems that arise from disability.

For persons with disabilities, the family presents the greatest source of physical, psychological, social and economic support. It is widely acknowledged that families and friends provide up to 90% of the care for people with disabilities who live at home (Peat, 1991) and that the support of informal networks, like families and friends, influences the final outcome of rehabilitation. Although families have the major responsibility of caretaking for the family member with a disability, they rarely receive the needed support from the wider community. Families need support in the areas of education, liaison with other organizations, social interactions, technology, economic and social problem solving and information sharing.

Costs to Society

Studies have consistently found that disabled people as a group are poorer, and have fewer years of school, fewer occupational skills, more unemployment and higher rates of poverty. The life situation of persons with disabilities can be described by a reduced level of performance, lack of income and employment, and exclusion from participation in the community. The costs and burdens of disability are very great and are borne by many statutory and non-statutory services as well as by individual people. The burden is particularly high in terms of money, manpower and equipment. To these direct costs should be added the loss of potential income for disabled people and the contribution they could make to community life and the generation of wealth (Peat and Boyce, 1993).

Poor community rehabilitation services increase the number of hospital admissions resulting from accidental injury, from avoidable infections, the development of avoidable deformities and from stress-related disorders. The length of stay in a hospital after injury or after disabling illness, such as stroke, is often inappropriately prolonged by the lack of effective continuing care at home or by delays in adapting the home and community environments (McLellan, 1992).

The Need for Change and the CBR Solution

Keeping disabled people in dependency is costing many times more than would helping them to independence. To do nothing now, on the basis that our ability to respond to the problem is constrained by inflation is to feed that inflation and further reduce our capacity to solve the problem of disability. The costs of not eliminating dependency will vastly exceed the cost of spending to make the disabled independent. (Bowe, 1980)

In order to address the problem of disability, it is necessary to:

♦ expand research and technology transfer efforts to prevent, cure and ameliorate the effects of ageing and disability;
♦ remove architectural, transportation,

and communication barriers facing disabled and elderly people;

♦ increase efforts to train disabled and elderly people;

♦ reform dependence-oriented policies and programmes.

To this end, persons with disabilities are taking a major role in advocating for change and are organizating themselves in ways that give them a stronger voice in influencing local and national governments, and the international non-government sector.

Awareness Building and Self-organizing

Persons with disabilities began sharing their personal experiences and realized that they faced many of the same problems regardless of the disability. They became aware that their problem was not in the disability itself but in the community that excluded them from the mainstream and deprived them of basic human rights. The movement of persons with disabilities has been seen by them as a second civil rights movement (Driedger, 1989). Pioneers of this movement saw persons with disabilities as citizens with civil rights, as people with human rights and as consumers with power in the marketplace. They rejected the role of the patient and client and transformed themselves into the empowered members of their communities (Arsenault, 1993). They identified the professional–client relationship, as well as environmental and attitudinal factors, as the most significant barriers to access and equality (Lysack and Kauffert, 1993).

Persons with disabilities realized that they needed to regain their self-esteem and create a new and more positive image of a person with disability. As the community sends mostly negative messages about the inferiority of persons with disabilities, the process of developing self-esteem may be long and frustrating. However, a positive image of a person with a disability with high self-esteem influences the attitudes of society and the community. As long as the person with a disability is viewed as the problem, the disabling factor of negative social attitudes will not change.

WHAT IS EMPOWERMENT?

Empowerment is a process in which an individual or a system is given power or authority (Oxford English Dictionary, 1978). It comes through participation in decision-making in important issues that influence everyday life (Coleridge, 1993). For persons with disabilities, empowerment means self-direction and self-determination. Instead of permitting health professionals to determine their interaction and participation, persons with disabilities are encouraged to take control over their lives.

Empowerment is a feeling of self-worth that comes from the awareness of one's own value and from having an influence over one's life (Coleridge, 1994). Empowerment is a mindset. People can be technically empowered but unless they consider themselves to be empowered or feel empowered, they are not empowered (Emener, 1991). People must believe that they are entitled to take control over their own lives to be able to do so. Empowerment is a two-way process between the community and persons with disabilities. All are enriched in this process because another's development and independence enriches all components of society. Empowerment of persons with disabilities and communities is achieved through their participation as partners working on issues such as primary health and social care and rehabilitation and advocacy. It has changed power relationships between groups of persons with disabilities and well established professional groups and rehabilitation organizations (Lysack and Kauffert, 1993).

The term empowerment is often associated with CBR. The main elements leading to empowerment are greater individual choice and public participation in the rehabilitation process. The choices that people make are greatly influenced by a number of variables, such as demographics or cultural factors. It is also known that well informed communities make better decisions. Achieving empowerment of the individual begins with strengthening the democratic process of health care. CBR should be considered a process of democratizing rehabilitation, making it more accessible to persons with disabilities.

There are four factors in two areas of empowerment that are critical to rehabilitation service delivery. The following descriptive framework is based on an empowerment approach to rehabilitation service delivery developed by William Emener in 1991. Important internal and external considerations and illustrations of empowerment are included in the following four areas:

- rehabilitation systems (agencies, companies, facilities);
- rehabilitation professionals (counsellors, managers, administrators);
- families of persons with disabilities (or caregivers);
- persons with disabilities.

Rehabilitation Systems

Critical factors in two areas of system empowerment

External empowerment	Internal empowerment
Laws	Organizational
Negotiations	philosophy
External systems	Policies and procedures
management	Competent staff
Image control and	Leadership style
marketing	
Efficiency and	
effectiveness	

External

As the world and society continues to change, the field of rehabilitation and rehabilitation systems must continuously and proactively change (McDanial and Jacobs, 1981). It is essential for proposed and active public laws and policies to 'empower' systems, which is to say that the system should be given control over the development and implementation of effective and efficient services for persons with disabilities.

Internal

Organizational philosophy, policies and procedures should be designed and managed in a way that permits a system to empower itself to achieve self-direction, self-improvement and self-governance. For example, rehabilitation professionals become frustrated when the systems in which they work do not accommodate their need for freedom and autonomous functioning. It is not only important for rehabilitation systems to be empowered, it is also important for them to be designed and managed in ways that facilitate the empowerment of the professionals working within them.

Professional

> ### Critical factors in two areas of professional empowerment
>
> | External empowerment | Internal empowerment |
> |---|---|
> | Competency | Competency |
> | Efficiency and effectiveness | Knowledge and skills |
> | Professional sanctions | Professional self-concept |
> | Negotiations | Collegiality |
> | Image control and marketing | Networking |

External

In order to be assured of empowerment, rehabilitation professionals must be competent. Demonstrating high level skills, and efficient and effective service delivery, is important to establishing and maintaining a desirable public image.

Internal

Internal self-empowerment of rehabilitation professionals is also important. Self-empowered professionals have more positive attitudes, a higher level of job satisfaction, perform better and promote self-empowerment of persons with disabilities. The self-concept of professionals and their sense of collegiality and networking is critical to their career and professional endeavours and the extent to which they are empowered as professionals.

Families

> ### Critical factors in two areas of family empowerment
>
> | External empowerment | Internal empowerment |
> |---|---|
> | Economic security | Communications |
> | Family management | Individual competency |
> | Functional effectiveness | Individual input |

External

The family is of paramount importance to the successful rehabilitation of persons with disabilities. External empowerment of the family occurs when appropriate levels of assistance are available that contribute to the economic security of the family unit. Often family members are more supportive of persons with disabilities than rehabilitation professionals, thus families should be assisted to manage themselves.

Internal

Families should be encouraged and assisted to empower themselves to prevent and overcome difficulties that individual family members have, as well as the difficulties that present themselves to the family as whole. Families need to achieve a healthy balance between meeting the needs of the person with disabilities and the overall needs of the family.

Persons with Disabilities

> ### Critical factors in two areas of empowerment of the persons with disabilities
>
> | External empowerment | Internal empowerment |
> |---|---|
> | Economic security | Individual competency |
> | Effective living | Healthy self-concept |
> | Lifestyle management | Meaningful relationships |
> | | Networking |

External

External empowerment for persons with disabilities exists when the individual is provided with adequate economic security and appropriate social networking which permits them to govern their own lives. In teaching effective life skills to individuals with disabilities, it is important to include topics related to lifestyle management and self-management.

Internal

Individuals with disabilities must empower themselves, by conceptualizing self-empowerment from an internal perspective. Once a person with disabilities has developed a strong self-concept, meaningful interpersonal relationships and supportive social networks, they are in a position to empower themselves.

CHARITABLE ORGANIZATIONS

In the 1970s the primary model for programming for persons with disabilities was the medical rehabilitation model. This model viewed persons with disabilities as passive recipients of care and unable to participate fully in community life in the same way as non-disabled persons. Persons with disabilities remained hidden in the seclusion of special rehabilitation institutions or their homes where rehabilitation treatment could be provided to them. The special institutions for caring for those disabled by severe neurological deficit or leprosy are examples of the removal of persons with disabilities from the community. The main goal of the medical model for physical rehabilitation was to help persons with disabilities adapt to the physical limitations of everyday life. This approach inadvertently encouraged their exclusion by maintaining the 'status quo'. Consequently, people with disabilities have felt isolated and marginalized, and unable to participate because of environmental and attitudinal barriers.

Many charitable organizations developed programmes for persons with disabilities in order to ease the burden of disabilities. However, this support model was based on 'helping' and not on the 'empowering' of individuals to take responsibility for their own lives. These organizations did not change the status of persons with disabilities but made them even more dependent on the compassion and sympathy of 'good people'. Persons with disabilities were not regarded as equal members of the community but as a group that deserved pity from all those who were not disabled.

ORGANIZATIONS OF PERSONS WITH DISABILITIES

A major feature in the global rehabilitation environment in the last twenty years has been the emergence of organizations, nationally and internationally, which represent the needs and aspirations of persons with disabilities and their families. Historically persons with disability had not organized themselves socially or politically. The period of major growth in the development of organizations of persons with a disability was between 1965 and 1970. These organizations were particularly successful in economically advantaged societies where they exerted a great deal of influence over the allocation of resources for rehabilitation services, and the development of public policy in relation to disability issues.

Organizations representing the needs of persons with disabilities identified a number of objectives including:

+ improving the status of persons with disabilities;
+ promoting self-help by persons with disabilities;
+ providing a democratic structure through which persons with disabilities could voice their concerns and opinions;
+ monitoring public policy and legislation;
+ promoting policies determined by persons with disabilities;
+ sharing information with international organizations of persons with disabilities to establish a positive image of persons with disabilities. (COPOH, 1991).

Prior to the successful establishment of organizations such as COPOH, many charitable organizations worked for disabled people and tended to focus on disability issues which reinforced the concept that disabled persons were unable to perform in an environment made for non-disabled people. The founders of the disability movement realized that the charitable and medical model approach was incapable of addressing the social and physical barriers which disabled people found in society.

Organizations for persons with disabilities saw their role as:

♦ vehicles for public education;
♦ lobbying for changes to environmental barriers;
♦ evaluating and monitoring services;
♦ encouraging membership development;
♦ advocates of human rights legislation, including physical access and transportation.

At present there are four primary organizational structures of persons with disabilities: consumer organizations, advocacy groups, the independent living movement and self-help groups.

Consumer Organizations

Consumer organizations take part in the political life of society because without political determination and commitment to change little can be achieved. In order to have a greater influence in the political discourse, the structure of these organizations follows the political and administrative organizational structure of society.

Local Level

A network of local organizations, using flexible and informal structures, aims to involve the entire membership in planning and implementing strategies. This total involvement enables the process of empowerment of its members. Regional organizations have the geographic scope and jurisdictional mandate to unite the wide range of groups of persons with disabilities.

National Level

The main purpose of a national organization is to focus on major national human rights legislation, and legislation which affects the allocation of funding and policy in areas of vital importance to persons with disability. The areas of particular interest to persons with disabilities are transportation, housing, education, employment, social security, rehabilitation services and independent living support systems (Gadacz, 1994).

An example of a national consumer organization is the All Russia Society of the Disabled (ARSD). This is the only national organization of physically disabled people in Russia. It is directed and administered by persons with disabilities and comprises 2.2 million individual members affiliated through 78 regional member organizations, 444 420 district and city organizations and over 19 000 local member organizations. Each regional and district ARSD organization has its own legal constitution and board.

International Level

Disabled People's International (DPI) is the first successful effort of persons with a disability to create a united voice in the international forum. DPI was established in 1981 in Singapore and currently has an active membership in over 100 countries around the world. The constitution accepted in Singapore asserted the basic rights of persons with disabilities as participants in society having the right to education, rehabilitation, employment, independent living and income security.

Members of DPI assert a shared conviction that persons with disabilities must have a voice to express their priorities, and a movement through which to take action. Attainment of these goals will lead persons with disabilities to a life of full participation and equalized opportunities.

While DPI is respected as a grassroots catalyst for change, equally important is the fact that it is also the sole international representative of the unified voice of persons with physical, mental and sensory disabilities. DPI's presence in international operations is strong. DPI has collaborated with the United Nations Economic and Social Council Organization, the World Health Organization and the International Labour Organization. Recently DPI worked closely with the United Nations in the development of the UN World Program of Action Concerning Disabled Persons. In this collaboration, DPI and UN agencies attempted to implement the shared principles of self-determination, full participation and equalization of opportunity for persons with disabilities.

DPI is a development organization whose main function is to foster and encourage the development and liberation of its members. It is not an operational agency nor a funding agency. It is an organization established by its members to foster the development of a worldwide membership and to animate persons with disabilities to take charge of their lives. The development programme operates within a backdrop of acquiring the facilities, infrastructure and the financial resources necessary to enable and to empower its membership to assume control over the forces that has led to their underdevelopment.

Major functions of DPI
Communication:
♦ Facilitate information flow.

♦ Communicate with UN and other international agencies.
♦ Publish Vox, Nostra, DPI Newsletter.
♦ Publish and distribute information and annual reports.

Research and analysis:
♦ Evaluate development programmes.
♦ Develop research centres.
♦ Research issues of concern to disabled people.
♦ Analyse policies and practices that affect disabled people.

Organization, support and maintenance:
♦ Organize meetings re: DPI.
♦ Conduct regional and world assemblies.
♦ Assist with local fundraising.
♦ Nurture worldwide membership.

Monitoring, advocacy, public attitude change:
♦ Pursue improved human rights.
♦ Seek change in policies/practices of UN.
♦ Implement DPI World Programs of Action.
♦ Increase and enhance involvement of disabled people.
♦ Develop and carry out activities which enable disabled people to represent themselves.

Self-help movement development:
♦ Encourage and assist new self-help groups.
♦ Identify regional development needs.
♦ Raise funds for development programmes.
♦ Develop and distribute resource materials.
♦ Facilitate projects that enhance socio-economic opportunities.
♦ Foster international experience exchanges.
♦ Monitor and evaluate programmes and projects.

The DPI self-help development programme seeks to increase the participation of disabled people in the social and economic development of their countries and communities. Of particular concern to DPI is the status of women with disabilities and refugees with disabilities living in rural areas. Through DPI their voice has already been heard not only in regard to disability concerns, but also on issues of justice, human rights, peace and international development (DPI, 1995).

Another example of an agency working at the international level is the World Institute on Disability (WID) which was founded in 1983 and operates from a base in Oakland, California, USA. WID is a public policy, research and training centre dedicated to independence and equal opportunity for all people with disabilities. This organization is committed to:

♦ empowering persons with disabilities to take control of their own lives;
♦ challenging attitudes that stereotype people with disabilities;
♦ changing public policies that keep persons with disabilities dependent at home or in institutions;
♦ teaching people with disabilities to define and communicate their own desires and needs;
♦ educating the public, policy-makers, business and the media about people with disabilities and independent living;
♦ training the future leaders of the independent living and disability rights movement.

WID works with a variety of constituencies: people with disabilities, parents of children with disabilities, disability organizations, government and private policy-makers, corporations, foundations, academia and the media. Because of its extensive collection of information on personal assistance services, WID is con-tacted by people from around the world for information and ideas. WID's projects include education and training, AIDS and disability awareness, personal assistance experiences, telecommunications and a variety of international programmes and initiatives.

WID is helping to create a future in which people with disabilities have equality of opportunity and where policies and services supporting independence are developed. Stereotypes that people with disabilities can't work and must be taken care of are challenged and replaced. The reality is that people with disabilities have unlimited potential – when barriers of attitude, architecture and policy are removed. (WID, 1996).

Consumer Groups and Community Based Rehabilitation

Consumer groups are very vocal in advocating for policy changes that promote equal opportunity. The following actions would result in the removal of or reduction to the barriers that exist for persons with disabilities.

♦ development of high quality, accessible rehabilitation (medical, vocational, education);
♦ flexible attendant care and interpreter services;
♦ progressive social attitudes and social assistance;
♦ barrier-free communities (transport, public buildings, facilities);
♦ access to assistive devices;
♦ equal employment and educational opportunities;
♦ removal of disincentives to employment of persons with disabilities;
♦ flexible, accessible and coordinated community services;
♦ accelerated efforts to focus reform on the needs of persons with disabilities

and to empower persons with disabilities to participate in developing solutions.

The following is a review of items that are on the agendas of consumer groups that also affect the implementation of CBR:

♦ attitudes toward disability;
♦ government policy;
♦ financial resource allocations of governments/agencies;
♦ personnel (knowledge and skills, roles and responsibilities);
♦ role of the consumer;
♦ service management and coordination;
♦ community environment: physical factors, demographics, infrastructure, technology, employment rate;
♦ community environment: social factors, values, morale, expectations, family support relationships.

Advocacy Organizations

The role of advocacy organizations is to monitor or assume the function of 'watchdog' over organizations that provide services (Arsenault, 1993). Three types of advocacy for persons with disabilities exist (Crichton *et al.*, 1994):

♦ system advocacy (restructuring social organization);
♦ support advocacy (actions of advocates on behalf of persons with disabilities);
♦ self-advocacy (persons with disabilities speaking for themselves).

System advocacy describes the organizations as well as the interactions of human service organizations and government services. Common targets of this type of advocacy would be schools, residential institutions, government services. Activities would include influencing public policy, initiating public education campaigns and promoting appropriate legislation.

Support advocacy includes associations or organizations that provide direct support to, and act on the behalf of, persons with disabilities and their caregivers and families.

Self-advocacy refers to people with disabilities who speak and act on their own behalf.

Independent Living Movement

The independent living movement, by challenging what and how services are provided, will continue to have an important impact on the cost of different services. The demand for medical and other professional services will decrease, and the demand for adapted housing and attendant care will increase. (DeJong, 1979)

The independent living movement was developed initially in the United States during 1960s and early 1970s. DeJong, an American disability advocate, suggested that the movement was inspired by the civil rights movement that sensitized society to the rights of disadvantaged groups and how their rights were being denied. In the same period, the independent living movement was born in Canada, with slightly different characteristics. Both North American models were the result of consumer-driven initiatives to assume control of lifestyle issues and so reduce the dominant influence of health and rehabilitation professionals. The development of independent living strategies was influenced by numerous factors including political and economic independence, development of medical technology, the emerging consumer movement and the self-help concept.

Activists in the independent living movement encouraged persons with disabilities to reject the patient role and to accept the role of consumer, to exchange the traditional institution based rehabilitation model with independent living in the community. This shift has led to a series of legislation changes by governments that have improved the position of persons with disabilities within their society. The rejection of the medical model of rehabilitation, deinstitutionalization and normalization are perceived as the three major factors influencing the development of the independent living movement (DeJong, 1979).

The Berkeley Independent Living Centre in California grew from the establishment of the Berkeley Independent Living Housing Venture which was developed by students with disabilities who realized that once they graduated, the services they needed to maintain an independent lifestyle such as attendant care and transportation would no longer be available. Three components were central to the Independent Living philosophy at Berkeley:

+ consumer control;
+ flexibility;
+ services which are responsive to recipients' needs.

The term 'independent living' has been used with different meanings depending on a variety of factors, including geographic location and political jurisdiction (Boschen and Krane, 1992). No matter how the movement is defined, it always has as its main goal the empowerment of persons with disabilities in order to remove social and environmental barriers that prevent them from controlling their own lives (Valentine, 1994). The definition of the term given by the first American Independent Living Centre, established in early 1970s in Berkeley,

California, is shown in the box below. This centre provided different services to persons with disabilities, such as transportation, attendant care, wheelchair maintenance, training in independent living skills, peer counselling and advocacy.

> **Defining the Berkeley Independent Living Model** (Frieden, 1980)
> Independent living is a program which is controlled by the disabled consumers it serves, and which provides services that are designed to assist people with severe disabilities to increase personal self-determination and to minimize unnecessary dependence upon others. The minimum of services that a centre for independent living must provide includes housing assistance, attendant care, readers and/or interpreters, peer counselling, financial and legal advocacy, and community awareness and barrier removal programs.

The history of independent living is based on the efforts of persons with disabilities who were seeking their rights in society. The values of the movement are consumer sovereignty, self-reliance, and political and economic rights. Consumers must rely primarily on their own resources and ingenuity to acquire the rights and benefits to which they are entitled.

Within the independent living movement the concept of Centres for Independent Living has emerged. These centres were organized to provide essential core services that include community needs assessment, interagency coordination, technical assistance, public information and education. The Canadian Association of Independent Living Centres (CAILC) promotes and enables citizens with disabilities to take responsibility for the development and management of personal and community resources (Boschen and Krane, 1992). Centres, while reflecting each community's unique character, are consumer controlled, cross-disability, non-profit, and promoters of integration and full participation. Essential programme components include information and referral, peer counselling, advocacy and service development capacity.

Independent living recognizes a person with a disability as an individual who has the same capacity and right to manage individual decisions, examine options, make choices, take responsibilities and risks, and make mistakes. From the community's point of view, the independent living movement encourages persons with disabilities to be equal citizens who fully participate in the life of the community while stressing their individual right of choice (Valentine, 1994).

Comparison of Community Based Rehabilitation and the Independent Living Movement

Community based rehabilitation (CBR) and independent living (IL) have a great deal in common. They share a broad definition of rehabilitation and encourage community participation while focusing on the needs of persons with disabilities. What differentiates the two is their governance and power structures. Where the principles of CBR foster community development on a partnership basis, IL encourages consumer control of all activities. This fundamental difference between CBR and IL makes them competitors in the development of rehabilitation strategies for the future (Lysack and Kauffert, 1993).

The independent living movement has its roots in North American societies. The focus of the movement has been shaped and directed by social and political environments. The common factor in health care in developed countries is the physician/professional dominance of the system. In Canada, as in European countries, social services and universal health care are in place, and food and shelter are generally adequate for its citizens. Consumers of services and persons with disabilities in these systems are free to scrutinize quality and the nature and availability of services without fear of being denied access to any health or social service.

Community based rehabilitation developed from much broader roots in a number of developing, economically disadvantaged societies where the majority of people receive limited or no rehabilitation services whatsoever. Disability identification, prevention of disability, early detection, provision of mobility aids and proper referrals are of primary concern. Although independence and empowerment are of importance in CBR strategies, and are of paramount importance to independent living, they may be perceived by communities in developing countries to be less important than receiving some direct and tangible service where none has existed before.

One of the fundamental aspects of CBR in economically challenged countries is the role of volunteers and community health workers. Independent living is 'for and by' persons with disabilities themselves and distinctly sees the involvement of non-disabled persons as leaning toward the charitable volunteerism of the past. IL, like CBR, relies heavily on volunteers, even though one of the main tenets of the IL movement is that the work of persons with disabilities should be recognized and valued by society. Both CBR and IL encourage positive attitudes towards persons with disabilities and the transfer of knowledge, skills and appropriate technology to communities and individuals. Both approaches motivate persons with a disability to become involved and empowered and to be the catalyst for change in their disabling environments.

Self-help Organizations

'A self-help organization of disabled persons is an organization run by self-motivated, disabled persons to enable disabled peers in their community to become similarly self-motivated and self-reliant' (Armstrong, 1993). They have been established for social, recreational or vocational reasons basically to meet the needs that are not met by other institutions in the society. Members of self-help organizations offer assistance to each other in the form of services/material assistance or advocacy. Not only do they lobby governments, influence national policies and programmes, they also provide rehabilitation aids and technology, housing and employment for their fellow members (Armstrong, 1993).

Self-help organizations and organizations representing the social and political aspirations of disabled persons can be regarded as having many similar objectives and strategies. Members of self-help organizations have the same mistrust of medical rehabilitation services as do the members of consumer groups. Like consumers, members of self-help groups tend to give persons with disabilities the opportunity and responsibility to make decisions on matters that affect their lives. They support each other in an effort to contribute to the well-being of their communities (DeJong, 1979). Self-help groups can focus on a single disability such as leprosy or multiple sclerosis or they can be cross-disability organizations as in the case of the Fiji Disabled People's Association. The emergence of self-help groups is a feature within the broader disability movement. In some geographical and social locations, the term 'self-help' has enjoyed greater social acceptance than the term 'consumer movement'.

UNI-DISABILITY AND CROSS-DISABILITY ORGANIZATIONS

As a result of the influence brought to bear by the medical approach to rehabilitation, the first organizations of persons with disabilities were *uni-disability* agencies, organized around one common disability issue such as visual or hearing impairment. Examples of this type of consumer group would be the Swedish Deaf Project, Sweden, the National Association of the Deaf, Thailand, and the Sri Lanka Federation of the Visually Handicapped. Individual groups found that they could achieve a stronger voice if they worked collectively, and that led to the establishment of *cross-disability* organizations such as the Handicapped Housing Society of Alberta (provincial) or the Coalition of Provincial Organizations of the Handicapped (COPOH) (national) or the Canadian Rehabilitation Council for the Disabled (national). These cross-disability organizations were established to overcome the consequences of a fragmentation in programmes related to disability. Joint action promised more benefits than could be achieved in separate ventures (Gadacz, 1994).

THE CONSUMER MOVEMENT

Consumerism embraces almost all social classes and groups, including disadvantaged groups, in society. Consumers want to get as much product or service as possible for the resources available and feel that it is their responsibility to be informed about the quality, adequacy and reliability of products or services. Consumers demand a clean and healthy environment, safe streets, better transportation, comprehensive health care and other services and goods that improve their well-being. Consumerism is characterized by a general mistrust of sellers or service providers. In consumer organizations, people have found that their collective voice and experience, and their collective strength can influence the marketplace and government mechanisms to respond more adequately to their needs.

Disability consumerism has been developed out of a basic need to make informed decisions about important issues of one's own life. It is a response to the traditional medical approach which neglects the involvement of an individual with a disability in the decision-making process and assumes that the person with a disability is 'sick' and unable to take responsibility for his or her personal affairs. In this approach, decisions about the lives of persons with disabilities and the treatment and services that are needed ought to be made by health professionals who are regarded by society as competent to do so. Consumers with disabilities have rejected this approach and role and have become personally involved in planning their treatment.

Persons with disabilities have organized consumer advocacy groups to influence the choice of services provided to meet their needs, to monitor the quality of products and services, to provide information about legal rights and entitlements, services, education, and research into developing technologies and available programmes and practices. These organizations do not usually provide technical services such as equipment and assistive devices, prosthetics, pharmaceuticals, transport systems, career training or housing. They offer legal advice and access to reference libraries, which enables persons with disabilities to be better informed about governmental benefits and regulations and possibilities to use them. Persons with a disability want services to be better coordinated, more efficiently managed, affordable,

equitable, universally accessible and consumer-driven.

The following issues have been identified by the consumer movement. These principles are used to inform government and professional agencies of those factors which could make society more accessible for persons with disabilities.

Self-determination
This principle suggests that persons with disabilities make their own informed decisions about lifestyle choices and that the choices that are made be respected.

Integration
This principle points out the right of persons with disabilities to use the same services and facilities which are available to other members of society.

Full participation
The participation principle means that persons with disabilities must have the same opportunity to participate fully in all the educational, employment, consumer, recreational, community and domestic activities which are part of everyday life of the society.

Independent living
This principle stresses that persons with disabilities must have the opportunity to manage and develop the disability services which they require in order to live independently in the community.

Consumer control
This principle articulates that persons with disabilities must have control of their self-representational organizations at the decision-making level.

Equality
This principle goes far beyond a model of equality, because equal treatment will not always assure the equality of results.

Equality implies the equalization of opportunities, as stated in the definition of the UN World Program of Action, through the process in which 'the general systems of society such as the physical and cultural environment, housing and transportation, social and health services, educational and work opportunities, cultural and social life, including sports and recreational facilities are made accessible to all' (D'Aubin, 1986).

ROLE OF WOMEN

Women play a major role in CBR; they are the nurturers in the family and most community workers are women. In the literature on CBR, where we read 'community' we should read 'family', and for 'family' we should read 'women' (O'Toole, 1987; Peat and Boyce, 1993). In developing countries, where a family member has a disability, women are the primary caregivers who dedicate their lives to providing care, very often neglecting their own needs and exposing themselves to the risk of becoming disadvantaged themselves. When addressing disability issues, gender is an important factor. As a result of studies, many recommendations have been made which suggest that the status of women must change, yet there are few concrete suggestions as to how this can occur. In developed countries, women are also the primary caregivers with little formal support from the community. One study concluded that because of the inadequacy of formal assistance, caregivers often must chose between placing a relative in an institution or carrying on at great personal cost (Callahan, 1988; Peat and Boyce, 1993).

The place of women with disabilities in society is significantly influenced by the position of women in society in general. Women with disabilities have been denied the opportunity of demonstrating their abilities to contribute fully to their communities. Discrimination against women can be very severe affecting all aspects of life such as education, employment, economic status, marriage, family and rehabilitation. Many women are being deprived of their rights and society is being deprived of the talents and abilities of women with disabilities, because of a lack of opportunity. In many societies, education of women is not a priority, and education for disabled women is even less of an issue. Because of the perceptions of the able-bodied, women with disabilities are often encouraged to channel their energies into hand work such as dressmaking, carpet weaving, and needlework, rather than recognizing that some women with disabilities may have an aptitude for business, management or professions (Fine and Asch, 1988).

In societies where women are oppressed, women with disabilities experience the same difficulties and challenges as other women, but suffer further disadvantage because they do not have the same position within society as able-bodied women. For this reason women with disabilities are considered to have a double disadvantage. In developing societies women are expected to carry the responsibility for the bulk of domestic labour including raising crops, providing water and fuel, home making duties and child care. CBR programmes in developing societies that rely heavily on the voluntary participation of the family must be sensitive to any unrealistic demands that additional responsibility may place on female family members (Peat, 1991).

Women with disabilities experience discrimination in education, the labour force, and at times, in their own families. Caring family members tend to overprotect a child with disability, especially girls. Accounts of the lives of disabled women and men reveal that boys are often more encouraged to meet the world whereas girls are more often kept from it. Class, race, ethnicity, and values of the parents and family and the medical professionals with whom they interact, powerfully influence the parental response to a girl with a disability (Fine and Asch, 1988). Franklin in 1977 reported that women with a disability were less likely than women without disability to be married, were more likely to marry later and were more likely to be divorced. Men and women with disabilities are poorer than those without disabilities. Women with disabilities are at the bottom of the economic ladder of society, fewer women than men with disabilities participate in the labour force and very often women are consistently unemployed or underemployed. Usually employed women with disabilities work in low wage service sector positions (Fine and Asch, 1988).

Women with disabilities encounter greater obstacles to marriage and child rearing. Women are often valued by a society that judges people in terms of physical appearance. If a woman becomes disabled after her marriage, she is at greater risk that her husband will leave her for another partner or that she may be judged incompetent to care for her children. Disabled women are commonly considered unfit as sexual partners and as mothers. 'Many women speak angrily of the unavailability of counselling on sexuality . . . from either gynaecologists or rehabilitation professionals. As disabled women it is doubly difficult for us to be accepted and our own sexuality discovered. The more obvious the disability, the more likely we will be thought of as asexual. Frequently, we begin to believe that we have no rights to sexual feelings. Women with disabilities traditionally have been ignored, not only by those concerned about disability, but also by those examining women's experiences. Perceiving disabled women as childlike, helpless and victimized, non-disabled feminists have severed them from the sisterhood in an effort to advance more powerful, competent and appealing icons' (Fine and Asch, 1988).

Despite the problems that disabled women and caregivers face in most societies, there are signs that more sensitive programmes are being developed. CBR, for example, has begun to recognize the needs of the mothers of disabled children. Through training programmes and the establishment of community support networks, CBR is offering some escape from the isolation that many women encounter. In developing societies some women do not view the problems of caring for disabled children to be their greatest concern. In their perception, what affects the family unit the most is poverty and the lack of community or family support.

In summary, CBR can play a major role in all societies in enhancing the qualify of life for persons with disabilities. In order to do so, it is essential that CBR works in partnership with the community of disabled persons to create an environment in which the disabled are empowered and regarded as equal and fully contributing members of society. It is only with this environmental change that the person with a disability will enjoy opportunities for employment and so contribute to the economic and social progress of their communities.

Barriers to successful CBR are the same as those faced by persons with disabilities in all their life experiences. CBR programmes work in partnership with communities for seeking to change the attitudes, beliefs and behaviours of health professionals, employers, and policymakers regarding the potential and ability of persons with disabilities. Until significant progress is made, there will continue to be economic penalties for people with disabilities and their families.

REFERENCES

Armstrong, J. J. (1993) Disability self-help organizations in the developing world; a case study from Malaysia. *International Journal of Rehabilitation Research* **16**: 185–194.

Arsenault, F. (1993) From Clients to Consumers: The Canadian Disability Rights Movement. Conference presentation, International Centre for the Advancement of Community Based Rehabilitation, Queen's University, Kingston, Canada.

Boschen, K. and Krane, N. (1992) A history of Independent Living in Canada. *Canadian Journal of Rehabilitation* 6(2): 79–88.

Bowe, F. (1980) *Rehabilitation America: Towards Independence for Disabled and Elderly People.* Harper and Row, New York, p. 283.

Callahan, D. (1988) Families as caregivers: the limits of morality. *Archives of Physical Medicine Rehabilitation* **69**: 323–328.

Coalition of Provincial Organizations of the Handicapped (1991) *A Voice of Our Own.* From COPOH, 926 Portage Ave., Winnipeg, Manitoba, Canada.

Coleridge, P. (1993) *Disability, Liberation and Development.* OXFAM/ADD, Oxford.

Coleridge, P. (1994) Community participation and empowerment of people with disabilities. In *Community Based Rehabilitation (CBR).*

Crichton, A., Jongbloed, L. and Lee S. (1994) *Disability Policies in Canada: An Overview.* Unpublished manuscript, pp. 268–298.

D'Aubin, A. (Ed.) (1986) *Defining the parameters of independent living.* Available from the Coalition of Provincial Organizations of the Handicapped, 926 Portage Ave., Winnipeg, Manitoba, Canada.

DeJong, G. G. (1979) *The Movement for Independent Living: Origins, Ideology and Implications for Disability Research.* Michigan State University Center for International Rehabilitation, USA.

Disabled People's International (DPI) (1995) Promotional brochure on DPI. DPI Head Office, Evergreen Terrace, Winnipeg, Manitoba, Canada.

Driedger, D. (1989) *The Last Civil Rights Movement. Disabled People's International.* Hurt & Company, London, UK.

Edmonds, L. J. and Peat, M. (1996) Community Based Rehabilitation (CBR) and Health Reform: Timely and Strategic. Presented at the First Mediterranean Conference on Physical Medicine and Rehabilitation. Israel, May, 1996.

Emener, W. G. (1991) Empowerment in rehabilitation – an empowerment philosophy for rehabilitation in the 20th Century. *Journal of Rehabilitation,* Oct/Nov/Dec, 7–10.

Fine, N. and Asch, A. (1988) Introduction: beyond pedestals. In *Women with Disabilities*: Temple University Press, Philadelphia.

Franklin, P. (1977) Impact of disability on the family structure. *Social Security Bulletin* **40**: 3–18.

Frieden, P. (1980) Independent living models. *Rehabilitation Literature* **41**: 169–173.

Gadacz, R. R. (1994) *Re-thinking Disability.* University of Alberta Press, Edmonton; pp. 121–135.

Hammerman, S. and Maikowski, M. (Eds) (1981) *The Economics of Disability: International Perspectives.* Rehabilitation International with United Nations, New York.

Helander, E. (1993) *Prejudice and Dignity: An Introduction to Community Based Rehabilitation.* United Nations Development Program, New York.

Jongbloed, L. and Crichton, A. (1990) A new definition of disability: implications for rehabilitation practice and social policy. *Canadian Journal of Occupational Therapy* 57(1): 32–38.

Lysack, C. and Kauffert, J. (1993) Some perspectives on the disabled consumers movement and CBR in developing countries. *Actionaid Disability News* 7(5): 1.

McDanial, R. H. and Jacobs, M. F. (1981) Administration of rehabilitation services in rehabilitation facilities. In W. G.

Emener, R. S. Luck and S. J. Smits (Eds) *Rehabilitation Administration and Supervision*. University Park Press, Baltimore, MD, pp. 187–204.

McLellan, D. L. (1992) The feasibility of indicators and targets for rehabilitation services. *Clinical Rehabilitation* **6**: 55–66.

O'Toole, B. (1987) Community-based rehabilitation (CBR): problems and possibilities. *European Journal of Special Needs Education* **2**: 177–190.

Peat, M. (1991) Community based rehabilitation – development and structure: Part 1. *Clinical Rehabilitation* **5**: 161–166.

Peat, M. and Boyce, W. (1993) Canadian community rehabilitation services: challenges for the future. *Canadian Journal of Rehabilitation* **6**(4): 281–289.

United Nations Educational, Scientific and Cultural Organization (UNESCO) (1978). *Economics of Special Education: Czechoslovakia, New Zealand, United States of America*. UNESCO, New York.

United Nations Expert Group Meeting (1977) *Socio-Economic Implications of Investments in Rehabilitation for the Disabled*. Geneva.

Valentine, F. (1994) *The Canadian Independent Living Movement: An Historical Overview*. Canadian Association of Independent Living Centres, Toronto.

World Institute on Disability (WID) (1996) Home page information on the worldwide web, 29 May, 1996.

chapter
ten

Research in
Community Based
Rehabilitation

INTRODUCTION

Rehabilitation programmes at the community level and rehabilitation services in the institutional setting are for the most part practice fields and traditionally have undertaken research as a secondary interest. Those actively involved in community based rehabilitation (CBR) – the consumer, clinician or manager – have given attention to the development of CBR and the documentation of subjective impressions, while research methodology has not been reviewed comprehensively.

A review of CBR literature demonstrates that the primary interests of CBR personnel are the application of programmes, the development of alternative service models, and the education and preparation of those actively contributing to CBR development and implementation. The development of CBR over the last fifteen years has had a major influence on public policy in relation to disability issues. However, these initiatives

have not stimulated the development of research initiatives in community based practice.

Rehabilitation as a concept is relatively new, although its ideas and approaches have been known for several centuries. Most of the progress in rehabilitation research, and the profession of rehabilitation, has developed since the end of the Second World War in 1945 (Helander, 1994). Some aspects of rehabilitation related to specific clinical topics, such as the management of neurological and orthopaedic disease, have been advanced by the disciplines of bioengineering and computer science. More recently, research effort has developed around technological advances, such as independent living systems using electronics and computer assistance. The development of orthotic and prosthetic devices has also been accelerated through the use of high technology. Computer technology has expanded the capacity for research, as well as the complexity and magnitude of the projects contemplated. Increasingly, to be effective, research projects need to involve interdisciplinary collaboration among sociologists, psychologists, political scientists, persons with disability and rehabilitation professionals. However, 'these encouraging tendencies notwithstanding, scientifically unfounded methods and practice based on limited subjective experience still abound' (Helander, 1994).

With a higher priority being given to the enhancement of the technological aspects of medical care, the development of rehabilitation related research has been limited. The costs of inpatient diagnostic and treatment procedures in areas such as coronary care, emergency medicine and cancer treatment have created an international financial crisis in health care and the question of what society can afford is central to all debates at this time. As rehabilitation departments have often become 'the last resort' for people with all types of disabilities and have been forced to deal with the issues of long-term disability, they have not been able to attract the strong political and social support that has been given to the higher profile health issues that tend to attract greater public interest.

In the last decade, the rehabilitation professions have been very successful in developing the human resource base required for productive research. Excellent rehabilitation scientists with the appropriate education and experience in research have advanced both the basic science and clinical science components of rehabilitation practice. The transition from practice oriented to research based rehabilitation has not had the same impact in the environment of CBR, as there are few opportunities for appropriately educated scientists who are dedicated exclusively to the pursuit of research.

WHO IS INTERESTED IN RESEARCH?

Research has often been seen as an inaccessible and elitist activity because of the perception that research is the prerogative of the university and higher educational environment. This has dramatically changed in recent years with evidence that effective and relevant research can be conducted at many levels. Research carried out by community members is as relevant to the advancement of CBR as research activities resulting from the interdisciplinary collaboration of university research scientists. Those interested in research and its application to CBR include the person with disability, the family member or caregiver, the CBR worker or manager and those responsible for the development of public policy. In addition, educators in CBR must believe that research is a critical component of their mandate.

THE GOAL OF RESEARCH IN COMMUNITY BASED REHABILITATION

The ultimate goal of CBR is to improve the *quality of life for persons with disabilities*. To achieve this goal CBR research must be relevant and timely and lead to practical applications. There are a number of principles in CBR that are pertinent to the research process (Boyce and Peat, 1995):

♦ *Community*. Prabhu and colleagues in 1993 recognized the importance of the *relationships* between individual families, and groups and 'societies' within that community. This principle suggests that research should consider the various actors and many influences on disabilities that exist in a community setting.

♦ *Diversity* and *validity of knowledge.* CBR recognizes the diversity and validity of knowledge held by persons in different disciplines. This suggests that knowledge from many areas including education, rehabilitation, policy, technology, health and social sciences be considered.

♦ *Methodology.* In community research, there are many issues related to methodological rigour. After years of controversy, most researchers now recognize that qualitative, quantitative and participatory approaches are all appropriate depending on the questions being asked, and on the type of data which are available.

Research which aims to explore new aspects of the personal experience of disability may benefit from a *qualitative* method using in-depth interviews or observation. Research which requires outcome indicators of CBR programme coverage and efficacy may be best performed with a *quantitative* approach utilizing survey information or secondary statistical data. Finally, research intended to change local conditions through CBR projects may be done most appropriately through a *participatory* action approach which uses disabled persons' involvement in the planning, implementation and evaluation of community activities. Case study methodologies often incorporate all three of these approaches.

DIFFICULTIES IN CBR RESEARCH

The aims of rehabilitation are:

♦ to help physical recovery;
♦ to encourage physical, psychological

and social adaptation to disability and handicap;
♦ to promote a return to independence and activities of daily living;
♦ to prevent secondary complications.

Factors making CBR research difficult include:

♦ spontaneous recovery;
♦ diversity of formal rehabilitation;
♦ informal rehabilitation;
♦ outcome measurement;
♦ funding limitations.

Spontaneous recovery
Regardless of whether they receive formal rehabilitation or not, many people recover.

Diversity of formal rehabilitation
The variety of professional input, methods used, and kind of service delivery provided are factors affecting research effectiveness.

Informal rehabilitation
Institutionally based rehabilitation is a part of care provided to persons with disabilities. Informal rehabilitation services are provided by caregivers at home, without monitoring or evaluation.

Outcome measurement
Because rehabilitation deals with physical, psychological and social aspects of persons with disabilities and their caregivers, the outcomes used to assess effectiveness must be multidimensional and extend beyond the clinical indicators commonly used in medical research. Appropriate outcome measurement is problematic and several questions should be asked of outcome measures used in this area:

♦ Have the measures been properly evaluated?

♦ Are validated measures used consistently and over similar follow-up intervals to allow comparison?
♦ Do the measures reflect the range of dimensions relevant to rehabilitation?
♦ Can changes in the measurement scale be translated into clinically and socially meaningful terms?

Funding limitations

Rehabilitation is a relatively new speciality and evaluation of its outcomes is not always easily and clearly achieved; therefore, CBR research does not always attract appropriate funding support.

The size and variability of spontaneous recovery, the heterogeneity of what constitutes rehabilitation, the various modes of its delivery and the breadth of aspects of health and social functioning over which rehabilitation aims to have an impact present formidable difficulties for the researcher.

Besides the factors listed above which influence CBR research, some other problems and weaknesses have been identified: the inadequate size of trial populations, lack or poor choice of controls, poor definition of therapy, inappropriate outcome measurement, inability to generalize results, and lack of cost information (Pollock *et al.*, 1993).

These principles have important implications for CBR research and are related to developments in research in other health and social sciences (Boyce, 1994).

♦ *Nature of knowledge.* Previously the goal of research was to obtain 'facts' about 'reality'. This assumes that an objective reality exists, which is independent of the researcher's biases, training and ability to observe and measure phenomena. It has been suggested, however, that 'facts' and 'reality' are not absolutes, and the role of the research is vital in the research process. This issue is important in the application of research in disability which has often included paternalistic notions of disabled persons.
♦ *Linking personal experiences with policy development.* It is important to relate individual and collective experiences and needs to decisions which influence resource allocations. In CBR research, information should permit a linking of the various dimensions of issues and an integration of information at both the private and public policy levels. These levels, or sources of information, include the individual, the family, the community and the state or society.
♦ *Ethics of research.* Prabhu and colleagues in 1993 stated that in a newer area, like CBR, research is essential and may even be considered as an ethical necessity. However, it is vital that persons with disabilities are not harmed and that resources are not wasted in CBR programmes. A second ethical issue involves the active participation of subjects in the research process (Prabhu *et al.*, 1993).

CBR RESEARCH TOPICS

In 1991, Murthy asked the question '(in CBR) – is there a need for research?' The CBR community should now believe that research is vital if development of CBR is to be sustained. Within the last five years there have been a number of research areas which have emerged. The following are some of these topics:

♦ understanding the needs of disabled people and their families;
♦ service related research;
♦ technology;
♦ disability prevention;
♦ attitudes and beliefs towards disability.

The research questions which are frequently asked regarding CBR services are:

♦ What effect will this service have?
♦ What will it cost?
♦ Is that what people want?
♦ What will happen if the service is not provided? (Wirz, 1996)

Those providing financial resources and other forms of support for ongoing CBR programmes and activities require answers to these questions.

To date, research into CBR has tended to be service-based where CBR practitioners have described different approaches to service planning and delivery. Oliver (1990) has reviewed research methodologies related to disability and the application of participatory research where the design must involve persons with disability. The participation in research by persons with disability is vital in the further advancement of CBR. Wirz (1996) stated that the boundaries between service evaluation and research can become blurred. However, it is vital, if CBR practice is to be commonly informed by good service evaluation, that service evaluations be objective and replicable. In other words, good service evaluation should adhere to research practices.

Helander (1994) proposed the following as priority research areas in rehabilitation:

♦ design and testing of interventions to change negative attitudes toward persons with disabilites;
♦ investigation into efforts to include persons with disabilities in mainstream programmes;
♦ disability prevention in relation to home or agricultural occupational accidents; and early psychosocial stimulation of children under five years of age;
♦ development of effective delivery systems for CBR.

The CBR research topics shown in Table 10.1 illustrate five major project areas with specific activities and methodologies in the development of research in CBR.

Table 10.1   CBR research topics (Boyce and Peat, 1995)

CBR research topics	Projects	Methodology
Psychosocial	Attitudes, beliefs, behaviours in disability, self-appraisals of disability	Survey ratings and interviews, story analysis, interviews, associative tests
Role of women	Time use, social support and impact of CBR	Participatory rural appraisal Survey ratings
	Women as caregivers	Interviews and action methods
	Women with disabilites	
Knowledge/skill transfer	Effectiveness of CBR education	Case studies, ratings, interviews
	Peer group support	Action methods
	Impact of information systems	Ratings, interviews, technical data
Non-government organization (NGO) relationships	NGO collaboration networks	Survey ratings
	NGO/donor/state relations	Interviews, case studies
	Community services	Survey ratings
CBR policy	National policy	Interviews, archival data
	Children's rights	Interviews, document review
	Policy development	Document review

Psychosocial Issues

Among the many factors affecting disability, probably the most persistent are the attitudes, beliefs and behaviours surrounding a person with a disability. The social environment in which a person with a disability lives has a direct and dramatic effect on their quality of life. Two major areas for research questions for psychosocial issues are:

♦ *Indigenous concepts of disability* – What are the culturally specific concepts of disability which may be powerful motivators for action and/or mediators in the relationships of individuals and the community?

♦ *Self-concepts in disability* – How do persons with disabilities perceive their lives? What coping mechanisms are used by positive role models? How can these resources be utilized in self-help programmes in CBR? A major priority is the application of research methodology to the understanding of attitudes, beliefs and behaviours in the area of disability. These important issues were addressed in an international study by the International Centre for the Advancement of CBR (Berry and Dalal, 1996).

Studies are needed which address the important variations of psychosocial factors across cultures – the complex organizing systems of shared values and actions that affect both the meaning of disability and the social environments in which persons with disabilites carry out their lives (Boyce and Peat, 1995).

Role of Women in CBR

Role overload
The topic of gender is a critical aspect in all development activities. In relation to disability, it is important to study how CBR projects can be structured to avoid role overload for women. The overload factor can be both physical and social–emotional for women and older female children who are caregivers. Differences between caregiving in urban and rural communities are also of significance.

Double disadvantage
A second focus of gender research is related to the 'double disadvantage' of women with disabilities. How does disability interact with, and compound, the role of women in both developing and developed societies? How can female children with disabilities have equal treatment in CBR projects, when they do not have equal status in their communities? Self-help programmes for women with disabilities could be studied to answer these questions.

Knowledge and Skill Transfer

Technical and clinical skills
Education and training are often key components of CBR programmes. These include the transfer of technical and clinical skills, information resources, and knowledge about disability and rehabilitation from professionals and experts to communities and individuals. Of primary interest to researchers is the effectiveness with which CBR achieves this transfer.

Partnership in education
Another important issue is the concept of 'exchange', or more equal bilateral relationship, between groups involved in CBR.

Educational strategies
Studies on the nature of professional education and re-education are necessary to improve the preparation of professionals to work in community settings (Boyce and Peat, 1995).

Non-government Organization (NGO) Relationships

NGOs and donors
Many CBR projects are conducted by NGOs which receive their mandate and funding from a wide variety of donors. This research area addresses the relationships between the NGOs and their donors. Donors can include governments, multinational agencies, other NGOs, individual donors and communities.

Universities and NGOs
Of particular importance are the research needs of NGOs and the relationships between NGOs and universities involved in CBR. It is necessary to optimize the scarce resources available for CBR; the research partnership between NGOs and university sectors can be productive and vital.

NGO goals for research
Specific research areas include (1) non-government–donor–government differences regarding goals, and (2) differences between NGOs and communities in operational practices. Another important area of study is the shift from NGO 'commitment' to 'functionality'. The goal of this research topic is to understand fully the operational dynamics of NGOs (Boyce and Peat, 1995).

Policy Analysis
While there is well established interest in the study of disability epidemiology, programmes and policies in industrialized countries, similar analyses in developing countries have not yet been undertaken, especially in relation to community based programmes and services.

Policy making process
The focus of research is the study of the policy-making process in disability and rehabilitation. Such policy analysis can contribute to a better understanding of the interests of all stakeholders in CBR and of the mechanisms which can fully involve persons with disabilities in the policy process (Boyce and Peat, 1995).

PARTNERSHIPS IN RESEARCH

Many research activities, and the sustainability of research within the framework of CBR, would be enhanced by the development of collaborative research partnerships. At a time when financial constraints are being felt in all sectors, it is imperative to encourage the sharing of experiences, knowledge and skills. Research should not be considered the mandate of only one sector, as productive research will result from partnership programmes between the NGO and university sectors, and among NGOs, universities and government agencies. The collaborative approach to research should also include project organizers and most important of all, persons with disabilities from the early stages of the development of a research programme when questions are posed, to the analysis and interpretation of the findings. Research in CBR must be relevant to the needs of persons with disabilities and must contribute to the improvement of their quality of life and integration.

Some research areas related to medicine, such as management of patients with spinal cord injury, myocardial infarct and gait disturbances, have developed quite favourably. Other areas in which there have been positive results include education and vocational training, and the development of independent living systems using electronics and computers. In addition, some interdisciplinary research has been successful due to the combined efforts of sociologists, psychologists, medical specialists and therapists working to a common goal.

RESEARCH IN LESS DEVELOPED COUNTRIES

Rehabilitation services have been established to some degree in most less developed countries. The lack of adequate resources is one of the biggest problems that impedes the development and provision of rehabilitation services. As research is cost intensive it is relegated to a low priority by governments and donors.

> **Rehabilitation research in the less developed countries is significantly underdeveloped because:**
>
> ♦ Research is a new specialty and is still dominated by charitable organizations that do not give many funds for research.
> ♦ Qualified researchers with dedicated time are lacking.
> ♦ Research funds are lacking (Helander, 1994).

In summary, in sustainable research strategies, each project benefits from data and methodologies developed from other projects. It is important that the results of research be shared in a 'user friendly' manner with those involved in the CBR process, so they can determine their relevance and application to the future development of CBR activities. Research activities must be seen as fundamental to the concept of partnership (Pollock *et al.*, 1993).

Research can be promoted through:

♦ training programmes for researchers;
♦ dedicated research funds;
♦ publication and dissemination of user friendly information;
♦ development of partnership research activities;
♦ active involvement of persons with disabilities and caregivers;
♦ identification of priority research areas:

REFERENCES

Berry, J. and Dalal, A. (1996) *Disability, Attitudes, Beliefs and Behaviours. Report on an International Project in Community Based Rehabilitation.* ICACBR, Queen's University, Kingston, Canada.

Boyce, W. (1994) Research and evaluation in community based rehabilitation: an integrated model for practice. In *Asia Regional Symposium on Research and Evaluation in CBR.* ICACBR and Action Aid, Bangalore, India.

Boyce, W. and Peat, M. (1995) A comprehensive approach to research in community based rehabilitation. *NU News on Health Care in Developing Countries* 9: 15–18.

Helander, E. (1994) Policies, planning and research in developing countries. In *Asia Regional Symposium on Research and Evaluation in Community Based Rehabilitation.* Bangalore, India. United Nations Development Program.

Murthy, R. S. (1991) CBR – is there a need for research? *Action Aid Disability News* 2(2): 17–20.

Oliver, M. (1990) Changes in thinking about disability. In J. Swain, V. Finkelstein, S. French and M. Oliver (Eds) *Disability Barriers, Enabling Environments.* MacMillan, London.

Pollock, C., Freemantle N., Sheldong, T. and Song, F. (1993) Methodological difficulties in rehabilitation research. *Clinical Rehabilitation* 7: 63–72.

Prabhu, G. G., Barnes, M. P., Mennon, D. K., Ojha, K. N., Jena, S. P. K., Kuman, T. C. S., Chander, S. and Hairharan, S. (1993) Symposium on Research and Evaluation in Community Based Rehabilitation – Summary Proceedings. *Action Aid Disability News* 4 (2, Supplement): 2–12.

Wirz, S. L. (1996) Where should research in CBR be directed in the next ten years? *Action Aid Disability News* 7 (1).

Policies, Strategies and Services

INTRODUCTION

Politics is about far more than what we all can get: it is also about what we owe each other . . . The values of community and solidarity have been undermined and ignored. (Throne Speech, October 1990)

There are numerous public policy issues that must be considered in the establishment and maintenance of community rehabilitation services. These issues focus on problems of establishing new programmes within an existing institutional system. The future challenge for rehabilitation is to redirect and restructure a system that will respond to the needs of persons with disabilities in ways which minimize institutionalization and maximize secure and stable home, family and community living (Peat and Boyce, 1993).

MAKING POLICY

According to Gerein and Bickenbach (1995), there are four principles that guide the development of all social and health policy: autonomy, democracy, respect for diversity and equality. Other background principles of policy development are the more contentious issues of universal access and the demedicalization of health. In relation to community based rehabilitation (CBR), the following are the policy issues and questions which need to be addressed:

- How does society address inequities in access and quality of service?
- Can it be assured that a coordinated system of service delivery will not become another layer of bureaucracy?
- How can a balance be struck between the need for a strong community, in-home support system, and the need for facility-based care?
- How should community services relate to secondary and tertiary rehabilitation and health care centres?
- How will referral rights between levels be negotiated?
- Will there be boundary problems between community rehabilitation services and other disability service programmes?

♦ On what basis will decisions regarding community resources be made?
- by degree of need in the community?
- by social need?
- by degree of community involvement?
- by the need for professional involvement and ownership?
♦ What cost sharing and staff sharing arrangements can be made with other providers to ensure efficient use of resources?
♦ How will priorities be established and resources allocated?
♦ How will cooperation affect professional and legal responsibilities?
♦ What level of rehabilitation technology is appropriate for community services? (Peat and Boyce, 1993)

The field of disability and rehabilitation services is large and complex. It is therefore particularly important to select targets against a set of clear priorities and objectives. In many countries, including those with complex and organized health and social systems, programmes and policies related to disability and rehabilitation issues have developed in a piecemeal fashion without central planning at national, regional or district levels (MacLellan, 1992).

PUBLIC PARTICIPATION IN THE DEVELOPMENT OF POLICY

Social policy shapes both the form and the content of all human services, and plays a major role in the provision of adequate and appropriate services for persons with disabilities and their families by providing the legal framework for the allocation of technological, human and financial resources. Policy is the official stance or framework of decisions that cre-

ates responsibilities and implementation plans in relation to these responsibilities. The aim of health and social policy is to set out the legal and administrative strategies necessary to permit the resolution of health and social problems that have been identified through a political process (Gerein and Bickenbach, 1995). This may result in either the development of universal programmes directed at the needs of people at an aggregate level or programmes targeted at a specific segment of the population. Traditionally, the development of health and social policy has not involved wide consultation with all stakeholders. Policies related to health and social programmes have been developed according to, and in conformity with, the political agenda of professional groups.

The general population of consumers must play an important role directly or indirectly in supporting and approving any significant policy change in the health care sector. Past experience has shown that the public generally does not receive appropriate information with which to make informed decisions. The population of elderly, isolated and disabled persons are particularly vulnerable to a lack of information. Comprehensive social consensus is important in determining which needs of disabled persons will be met publicly, and to what extent. In the area of outreach and community programmes for disabled and elderly persons, attention must be given to the development of information systems which will describe rehabilitation options, benefits and services. This is particularly important if decentralization of decision-making to regional authorities and increased involvement by consumers are to be important parts of rehabilitation service policy. Up to this time the method of informing the public has been inadequate and individuals have had to approach several agencies to arrange for community services or to obtain advice and information. Mechanisms for transmitting rehabilitation policy information are underdeveloped or absent, and processes for identifying the views of the public and using this information in decision-making have been lacking (Stoddart and Bearer, 1992; Peat and Boyce, 1993).

Community members expect to be involved in the determination of priorities and planning of community and social services. Similarly, community members seek a role in overall policy development about community services and resource allocations (Stubbins and Albee, 1984; Peat and Boyce, 1993). There are benefits for community rehabilitation services which consumer participation may facilitate. Prevailing cynical attitudes toward service provision and professionals may be modified, therefore providing a more positive and productive relationship (Peat and Boyce, 1993).

Strategies for community involvement include:

♦ *Information sharing*: this is the weakest form of involvement, but is also the essential base upon which higher levels are established.
♦ *Consultation:* occurs when service providers ask informed consumers about their views and needs.
♦ *Negotiation:* occurs when the service provider and consumer 'bargain' about whether the consumer will accept what is offered.
♦ *Participation:* occurs when the provider and consumer both share in deciding what is acceptable; however, issues of relative power and influence are not addressed.

Community participation is often viewed as a panacea for a variety of problems in community based services. While the trend toward participation may provide more accountability, efficiency and promotion of a positive relationship between the consumer and the service provider, it should not be viewed naively. There are potentially significant problems that have been experienced in the practice of community participation.[1]

In any community environment there may be major differences between the interests of consumers and providers. Consumers are usually interested in increasing access to services and improving responsiveness to specific disability issues. They are also often interested in receiving a holistic approach to service; however, consumer apathy in actually involving themselves in the planning and implementation of health and community services may indicate that these programmes are not considered essential to the consumer's daily life and are only important when the consumer is ill or in need (Peat and Boyce, 1993). Professionals working in the community are usually interested in prevention of physical and psychosocial problems. However, the preventive tools at their disposal are primarily physical and behavioural and are not able to address more structural causes of disability and ill health, such as poverty and illiteracy (Dunn, 1990; Peat and Boyce, 1993). Many rehabilitation professionals have an appreciation of this dilemma and those who ignore the realities risk increasing the distance between consumers and professionals, which only serves to impair their ability to continue to work together.

When consumers and professionals work together, they are still likely to have different views on their respective roles. Thus, role conflict is possible in

---

[1] A more detailed discussion on the strengths/weaknesses and dynamics of community participation is included in Chapter 3.

the clinical, organizational and policy aspects of community rehabilitation services. Professionals tend to perceive that they should control the clinical aspects, participate in the organizational features and only marginally be involved in political or resource identification considerations. Consumers, however, perceive that they too should participate in the clinical aspects, fully control the organizational features of activities and share in the political and resource considerations with their more influential professional colleagues.

Rehabilitation services have not developed in any coordinated way. The result in many societies is a fragmented and overly complex sector with gaps in some places and duplication in others. This lack of a coordinated approach to rehabilitation programmes means that resources are not used as efficiently as they could be. The factors which contribute to the fragmentation of services include:

♦ different funding programmes;
♦ inadequate planning;
♦ rapid growth of non-government organizations and/or the private provider sector;
♦ unregulated services;
♦ inequitable access to services.

STRATEGIC PLANNING PROCESS AND PUBLIC POLICY DEVELOPMENT

The development of a strategic framework will provide the basis on which rehabilitation policies will be implemented. An example of this approach was seen in the recent development of the Ontario government strategy for redefining rehabilitation needs and policies which included the following areas:

♦ service delivery;
♦ system design;
♦ service planning;
♦ human resources planning;
♦ standards;
♦ accreditation.

In the policy development process, individuals from different geographical regions, and representing different interest areas formed stakeholder working groups which met over a 12 month period. Participants were drawn from all sectors and included:

♦ consumers;
♦ advocates;
♦ professionals and professional groups;
♦ public and private service providers;
♦ academics;
♦ insurers;
♦ Workers Compensation Board representatives;
♦ District Health Council representatives;
♦ government agency representatives.

The Working Groups met to review and analyse the key characteristics and the dynamics of the rehabilitation sector from their respective perspectives on the issues. Six main issues for the reform of the rehabilitation sector emerged out of the Working Group's reports and feedback from regional 'round table' discussions. A series of broad recommendations was then developed on the six major policy areas which addressed specific issues and provided the course of action for implementation. The six areas are as follows (Ontario Rehabilitation Services Strategy, 1995).

Funding
♦ Eliminate duplication.
♦ Funds based on functional need not on the cause of disability.

Access
- Expand the pool of providers who make referrals.
- Increase community services.
- Expand the use of creative and appropriate technology.

Service coordination
- Establish a provincial body to coordinate research, planning, information sharing, public education, advocacy and database management.
- Ensure that clients have access to a team of service providers through a coordinator.

Education and training
- Develop a public education campaign to improve awareness of rehabilitation issues.

Research
- Identify priorities of rehabilitation centred research.
- Keep a provincial database of completed and ongoing research projects.
- stimulate research on consumer centred outcome measures.

Standards
- Develop common functional based criteria for access to rehabilitation services.
- Develop clear and enforceable guidelines for addressing conflict of interest as it pertains to individuals, professional practice and the business environment.

In summary, in this example, the goal of policy development in rehabilitation in Ontario, Canada was to enable people with temporary and permanent disabilities to achieve optimal recovery and reintegrate into the community, by improving intersectoral coordination, integrating funding mechanisms, redistributing resources, enhancing resources in some areas and by making the system more accountable.

Factors Influencing Policy Development

Most policy changes are incremental in nature – slight adjustments that are made to existing policies, often in response to furthering personal political agendas. All changes to existing policy affect the population it serves (Gerein and Bickenbach, 1995).

Recent international initiatives and national commitments have marked the entry into a new policy era – one in which ideally all people should have access to health and related services as a human right rather than a commodity. Health is perceived by governments and policymakers as a powerful lever for socioeconomic development and political stability. Recognition of the social and moral obligation to include even the most disadvantaged, such as persons with disabilities, is beginning to dominate policy discussions.

The process of developing policy occurs in five levels:

- international and multilateral level;
- national level;
- provincial, state or district level;
- the implementing agency level;
- community setting.

There are many external and internal factors that influence the development of policies which include but are not limited to the following:

- credibility and public satisfaction;
- general public opinion and the social and political climate or environment;
- securing support in the form of networking;

- political appropriateness of issues and the public perception of the policy-maker responsible;
- leadership and communication style (Queen's University, 1995).

Identification of Priorities

The process of policy formulation includes the identification of priorities, the development of the goals to be achieved through intervention, the identification of broad strategies for the pursuit of these goals, and the assignment of resources to carry them through. Policies take effect when presented in a variety of forms, from general written statements to formal legislation, regulations, bylaws and taxation.

Governments may be reluctant to embrace new and innovative policies, as politicians must consider that policies that fail to follow through with action attract public attention through criticism from the opposition and petitioning of interest groups. A suggested approach to explore new policy trends would be to develop trial projects, and from their evaluation be able to extrapolate the results to possible project costs to the system and outcomes that could be expected on a national scale (Helander, 1995).

The process of determining priorities for policy development is based on gaining an understanding of the magnitude of the problem. The identification of priorities for policies related to rehabilitation involves a review of:

- the incidence and prevalence of disability;
- data on the severity and duration of disability;
- the stressors that are brought to bear on persons with disability and their families;

- technology available to solve problems for persons with disabilities;
- effectiveness of the current use of technology;
- what gains would be achieved through training of technical and management personnel.

Community Based Rehabilitation and Policy Development

Conditions that contribute to the effective development of policies include:

- maintaining open channels of communications among all stakeholders;
- consulting broadly with outside sources;
- assigning specialists and nonspecialists to develop policy, permitting ideas to be evaluated on the basis of their inherent merit rather than on the basis of the status of the originator;
- knowing when to get involved and when it is best to rely on 'masterful inactivity';
- decentralized practices;
- an environment that is conducive to intellectual freedom and freedom of speech;
- preparedness for some degree of risk-taking;
- an environment where participatory decision-making is encouraged (Queen's University, 1995).

'Community based rehabilitation should be considered an element of social, educational and health policy at all levels, and central to the concept of decentralizing the public sector. As a national policy, CBR can be part of a country's action plan in favour of people of all ages who have any type of disability. At the community level, the policy of integration is implemented under the auspices of the community, which owns the programme and which gives a major role to people with disabilities and their families' (ILO, UNESCO, WHO, 1984). For many years, policy experts held the belief that rehabilitation needs would be met the best by extending existing institutional services. After 15 years of functioning under this system, a viable alternative approach, community based rehabilitation, was introduced and remains generally accepted today.

CBR emphasizes a process of building up solidarity and confidence between health workers and the communities they service, which is necessary to achieve the goal of public health care. CBR responds to persistent policy problems surrounding issues such as access and equity. CBR is usually linked to existing primary health care, community development and the social welfare system and serves as a bridge between community and institutional services. Development of policy statements and planning are difficult with community programmes which encourage self-reliance, as the participatory activities developed during the programme are not only hard to plan in detail in advance but are difficult to incorporate as a component that will continue in a predictable, recurring or routine manner (Helander, 1995).

Effective CBR requires governments to transfer programme responsibility and resources to communities so that they can provide the basis of rehabilitation; however, governments must still be involved by providing the 'backbone' of technological resources and administrative support, and by being responsible for national multisectoral policy and programme coordination. Without changes that decentralize responsibility for programmes to the community, projects may only be mechanisms which improve the efficiency of existing government rehabilitation services through

mobilization of community resources. There is also a need for governments to provide guidelines for external donors and non-government organizations (UNDP, 1991). CBR policy strategies and implementation measures include a standard set of items including information and research, planning, legislation and economic policies, coordination of work, and the organization of persons with disabilities.

GOVERNMENT POLICIES

Developed Countries
The political processes of policy-making differ from country to country since these more directly involve basic political structures. As a rule, unitary systems as seen in the United Kingdom are able to implement ideological change in policy more quickly than non-unitary or federal systems such as Canada and Australia (Gerein and Bickenbach, 1995). In federal governments, there is a constitutional division of policy-making powers between federal and provincial or state governments, and inevitable conflict between the levels of government has hindered the prospects of meaningful reform. On the other hand federal systems allow for the input of regional and local differences in the shaping of social policy.

In the United Kingdom, the Griffiths Report (1988) tried to deal with the fragmentation of services between health and social services by recommending that local authorities be responsible for all community care services (Gerein and Bickenbach, 1995). In Ontario, Canada, similar recommendations have been received by the provincial government from the Association of District Health Councils, proposing a delivery model that would coordinate budgetary allocations and planning functions for existing services and agencies, through health units (ADHCO Long Term Care Bulletin, 1992).

Although more and more governments are developing policy statements which recognize the appropriateness and viability of community services for both economic and social reasons, there are difficulties with the logistics and administration of collaborative partnership between locally initiated projects and national service providers. However, community level participation determines the success of service delivery programmes in reaching the target populations or intended beneficiaries. Programmes that are most effective are those where there is a distribution of economic and political resources at the community level.

NON-GOVERNMENT ORGANIZATION POLICIES

Many consumers feel that despite government changes, they are still at the mercy of the system to some degree, including its inefficiencies and bureaucratic impenetrability. For this reason many consumers and professionals have organized into non-government agencies to provide what they feel the government does not, and in some cases to circumvent the various problems associated with government services. These non-government organizations prepare policy documents for their members and adherents which establish goals and strategies to achieve these goals. Many non-government agencies operate as independent entities, while others receive funding from government in whole or in part. For this reason, non-government organizations maintain good relations with government agencies, and keep at arm's length from political

radicalism in their policies and strategies (Bickenbach, 1993).

Non-government agencies tend to be less bureaucratic because they tend to be smaller organizations, but do have policies that guide their project activities. Implementation of activities is not as much of a 'top-down' process as it is in government programmes. Examples of non-government organizations include the World Blind Union, World Federation of the Deaf, CARE and Save the Children.

MULTILATERAL INTERNATIONAL DEVELOPMENT, GOVERNMENT AND NON-GOVERNMENT COLLABORATIVE POLICIES

Governments and multilateral agencies tend to be larger scale bureaucracies that have developed sophisticated organizational structures and administrative processes. Policy documents have been developed by many international development agencies. Of particular importance to the advancement of CBR and issues relevant to persons with disabilities is the UN Resolution Adopted by the General Assembly 48th session, Agenda No. 109, which incorporates a recommendation for governments to follow related to policy development and planning.

States will ensure that disability aspects are included in all relevant policy making and national planning . . . States have a responsibility to create the legal bases for measures to achieve the objectives of full participation and equality for persons with disability . . . States have the financial responsibility for national programs and measures to create equal opportunities for persons with disabilities. (UN, 1983)

The United Nations declared 1981 the *International Year of Disabled Persons* and 1983–1992 the *International Decade of Disabled Persons.* The United Nations General Assembly adopted the World Program of Action Concerning Disabled Persons. This detailed document provided a comprehensive description of potential components of national programme policy. In 1993, the United Nations General Assembly adopted the Standard Rules of Equalization of Opportunities for Persons with Disabilities.

Other policy developments of note in the past decade include (1) the International Labour Organization Convention No. 159 and (2) United Nations Recommendation No. 168 on Vocational Rehabilitation and Employment of Disabled Persons in 1993 on the subject of Equitable Training and Employment Opportunities for Disabled Persons. In 1994, a Joint Position Paper entitled *Community Based Rehabilitation for and with People with Disabilities* was published by ILO, UNESCO and WHO with the purpose of clarifying for policy-makers and programme managers the objectives of CBR and the methods for implementing it. It was hoped that this position paper would encourage governments and non-governmental organizations to review what had been accomplished by CBR in disability policies and to integrate CBR into community development.

A BRIEF COMPARISON OF GOVERNMENT AND NON-GOVERNMENT ORGANIZATIONS

The philosophy and approach to planning and implementing non-government (NGO) programmes are somewhat different from national health programmes. Initiatives for community participation activities undertaken by NGOs tend to emerge as a joint venture of NGOs and people. Projects of NGOs are often more locally oriented than government programmes and are not concerned when their activities do not align with national policies. The advantage of NGOs is that they do not preclude communities from organizing themselves to make requests related to their specific needs from the national system. Governmental and large multilateral agencies often experience political and bureaucratic pressures related to time frames, accountability and cost-effectiveness. With these procedures as the primary focus, there is little opportunity to develop community responsibility and ownership of programmes, or to obtain meaningful input from the community. Including community input in government programmes may reduce the value of the bureaucratic procedures.

HUMAN RIGHTS POLICY

The disability movement has often been seen as a human and civil rights movement, organized primarily to press for the adoption of basic human and civil rights legislation. Accessibility and equal opportunities are major concerns. Public transport has been seen as an important human rights issue closely related to economic self-sufficiency. Public services, housing, recreational facilities and schools must be accessible for all. If it is not possible to offer required services through regular community or private delivery systems serving the general population, persons with disabilities have proposed parallel systems as part of a transitional strategy. However, the concept of establishing parallel services for persons with disabilities retains some measure of discrimination and stigmatization.

Marginalization, discrimination, isolation, abuse, stigmatization are words commonly used to describe the position of persons with disabilities within their societies. There are many examples of physical, psychological, sexual and economic abuse of persons with disabilities. Because persons with disabilities are often denied their basic human rights, human rights have been the subject of attention in many international government and non-government organizations as well as in the United Nations. In 1993, the UN General Assembly adopted a set of Standard Rules on the Equalization of Opportunities for Persons with Disabilities in order to ensure that persons with disabilities may exercise the same rights, freedoms and obligations as other members of their societies. The Rules have been developed on the basis of experience gained during the United Nations Decade of Disabled Persons (1982–1993). Although the Rules are not compulsory, they imply a strong moral and political commitment to take action for the equalization of opportunities for persons with disabilities. In the Rules the term 'equalization of opportunities' is defined as 'the process through which the various systems of society and the environment, such as services, activities, information and documentation, are made available to all, particularly to persons with disabilities'.

The principle of equal rights implies that the needs of every individual are of equal importance, that those needs must be made the basis for planning in societies and that resources must be employed in such a way as to ensure that every individual has equal opportunities for participation. Persons with disabilities are members of society and have the right to remain within their local communities. They should receive the support they need within the existing structures of education, health, employment and social services.

However, as persons with disabilities achieve equal rights they should also have equal obligations. As those rights are being achieved, societies should raise their expectations of persons with disabilities. As part of the process of equal opportunity, provision should be made to assist persons with disabilities to assume their full responsibility as members of society.

The Standard Rules (United Nations, 1994), explained in detail in a recent UN publication, cover the following areas:

1. Awareness-raising
'States should take action to raise awareness in society about persons with disabilities, their rights, their needs, their potential, and their contribution.'

2. Medical care
'States should ensure the provision of effective medical care to persons with disabilities.'

3. Rehabilitation
'States should ensure the provision of rehabilitation services to persons with disabilities in order for them to reach and sustain their optimum level of independence and functioning.'

4. Support services
'States should ensure the development and supply of support services, including assistive devices for persons with disabilities, to assist them to increase their level of independence in their daily living and to exercise their rights.'

5. Accessibility
'States should recognize the overall importance of accessibility in the process of the equalization of opportunities in all spheres of society. For persons with disabilities of any kind States should

(a) introduce programmes of action to make the physical environment accessible; and (b) undertake measures to provide access to information and communication.'

6. Education

'States should recognize the principle of equal primary, secondary and tertiary educational opportunities for children, youth and adults with disabilities, in integrated settings. They should ensure that the education of persons with disabilities is an integral part of the educational system.'

7. Employment

'States should recognize the principle that persons with disabilities must be empowered to exercise their human rights, particularly in the field of employment. In both rural and urban areas they must have equal opportunities for productive and gainful employment in the labour market.'

8. Income maintenance and social security

'States are responsible for the provision of social security and income maintenance for persons with disabilities.'

9. Family life and personal integrity

'States should promote the full participation of persons with disabilities in family life. They should promote their right to personal integrity, and ensure that laws do not discriminate against persons with disabilities with respect to sexual relationships, marriage and parenthood.'

10. Culture

'States will ensure that persons with disabilities are integrated into and can participate in cultural activities on an equal basis.'

11. Recreation and sports

'States will take measures to ensure that persons with disabilities have equal opportunities to recreation and sports.'

12. Religion

'States will encourage measures for equal participation by persons with disabilities in the religious life of their community.'

13. Implementation and research

'States assume the ultimate responsibility for the collection and dissemination of information on the living conditions of persons with disabilities and promoting comprehensive research on all aspects, including obstacles which affect the lives of persons with disabilities.'

14. Policy-making and planning

'States will ensure that disability aspects are included in all relevant policy-making and national planning.'

15. Legislation

'States have a responsibility to create the legal bases for measures to achieve the objectives of full participation and equality for persons with disabilities.'

16. Economic policies

'States have the financial responsibility for national programmes and measures to create equal opportunities for persons with disabilities.'

17. Coordination of work

'States are responsible for the establishment and strengthening of national coordinating committees, or similar bodies, to serve as a national focal point on disability matters.'

18. Organizations of persons with disabilities

'States should recognize the right of organizations of persons with disabilities at national, regional and local levels. States should also recognize the advisory role of organizations of persons with disabilities in decision-making on disability matters.'

19. Personnel training
'States are responsible for ensuring the adequate training of personnel, at all levels, involved in the planning and provision of programmes and services concerning persons with disabilities.'

20. National monitoring and evaluation of disability programmes in the implementation of the rules
'States are responsible for the continuous monitoring and evaluation of the implementation of national programmes and services concerning the equalization of opportunities for persons with disabilities.'

21. Technical and economic cooperation
'States, both industrialized and developing, have responsibility to cooperate in and undertake measures for the improvement of the living conditions of persons with disabilities in developing countries.'

22. International cooperation
'States will participate actively in international cooperation concerning policies for the equalization of opportunities for persons with disabilities.'

Governments of the member states are encouraged to take greater responsibility in improving the position of persons with disabilities and implementing the Rules.

REFERENCES

ADHCO Long Term Care Bulletin (1992) *Planning a More Coordinated System*. Association of District Health Councils of Ontario, Toronto.

Bickenbach, J. (1993) *Physical Disability and Social Policy*. University of Toronto Press, Toronto.

Dunn, P. A. (1990) The economic, social and environmental obstacles, which seniors with disabilities confront in Canada. *Canadian Journal of Community Mental Health* 9(2): 137–150.

Gerein, N. and Bickenbach, J. (1995) Health and social policies. In *Physiotherapy for Older People*, Pickles (ed.). W. B. Saunders, London.

Helander, E. (1995) *Sharing Opportunities – A Guide on Disabled People's Participation in Sustainable Human Development*. Interregional Program for Disabled People. United Nations Development Program.

International Labour Organization (ILO), United Nations Economic, Social and Cultural Organization (UNESCO), and the World Health Organization (WHO) (1994) *Joint Position Paper on Community Based Rehabilitation for and with People with Disabilities*.

McLellan, D. L. (1992) The feasibility of indicators and targets for rehabilitation services. *Clinical Rehabilitation* 6: 55–66.

Ontario Rehabilitation Services Strategy (1995) *Strategic Priorities and Resources Group, Health Strategies Branch*. Ontario Ministry of Health, Kingston, Ontario, Canada.

Peat, M. and Boyce, W. (1993) Canadian Community Rehabiliation Services: Challenges for the Future. *Canadian Journal of Rehabilitation* 6(4): 281–289.

Queen's University (1995) *Rehabilitation Science 433 Management in Rehabilitation Therapy*. Course Outline. Kingston, Ontario.

Stoddart, G. and Bearer, M. (1992) Towards integrated medical resource policies for Canada: Information creation and dissemination. *Canadian Medical Association Journal* 147(9): 1325–1328.

Stubbins, J. and Albee, G. W. (1984) Ideologies of clinical and ecological models. *Rehabilitation Literature* 45(11–12): 349–353.

Throne Speech (1990) for the Province of Ontario, opening of the session in October, Toronto, Ontario, Canada.

United Nations (1983) *World Program of Action Concerning Disabled Persons*. United Nations, New York.

United Nations Development Program (1991) *Disabled People's Participation in Sustainable Human Development*. Division of Global and Interregional Programs.

United Nations (1994) Resolutions Adopted by the General Assembly of the United Nations. *Standard Rules on the Equalization of Opportunities for Persons with Disabilities*, 48th session, agenda item 109, New York.

World Health Organization (1981) Expert Committee on Disability Prevention and Rehabilitation, WHO Technical Reports Series, vol 68B, 7–37.

Conclusion

DECIDING THE FUTURE

Internationally there was a significant growth in the health and social sectors in the 25-year period from 1970 to 1995. This occurred at a time of major developments in the scientific and clinical base of rehabilitation practice. A major feature of this development has been the expansion of the institutional components of rehabilitation care and the development of specialization within the scope of practice of many rehabilitation professionals. The expansion of the institutional sector consumed a major proportion of the available financial and human resources to the extent that developments in other areas were constrained.

The development of the scientific and clinical base of rehabilitation occurred at the same time as the evolution of the consumer movement when persons with disabilities and their families became increasingly aware of their individual rights and needs. Also, within the last decade, many countries have become increasingly aware of their own limitations in providing the health and social services necessary to advance the rights of persons with disabilities. In the 1970s the medical and economic concepts of disability were challenged by persons

with disabilities organizations. Consumer groups became politically active in demanding equal opportunity and fundamental human rights. This created a new socio-political model of disability which stated that disability arose from the failure of the social environment to adjust to the needs of the person with disability rather than from the incapacity of persons with disabilities to meet the requirements of society (Jongbloed and Crichton, 1990).

The goal of community programmes is to enable a person with a disability to establish and maintain a lifestyle in which they enjoy equal access to social, cultural and economic privileges and opportunities. In some cases, the greatest barriers to community living and acceptance are the attitudes and beliefs toward disability prevalent in the population. Negative reactions, stereotyping and misconceptions remain major stumbling blocks to the successful operation of community based programmes. However, placing the responsibility for rehabilitation within the community can have a positive impact on the integration of persons with disability and can create a greater understanding of disability issues. In many societies there is now greater appreciation of the fact that persons with disabilities possess the talents, skills and capabilities to be active and productive in the community and competitive in the workforce.

Consumers can contribute to improved health and health care by:

- taking advantage of opportunities to be personally responsible for
  - making healthy choices in lifestyle;
  - preventing disability;
  - being informed about treatment options;
  - being aware of costs to the system;
- acting on behalf of communities for improved environmental, social and economic policies affecting health and the health care and social systems.

These consumer responsibilities must be balanced with equal effort and commitment on the part of regional and national governments. It is vital that the consumer be adequately informed in order to contribute effectively in the development of public policy. Therefore, access to information together with public education programmes will enable communities to make better choices. (Ontario Ministry of Health, 1989).

Strategies must be implemented that will facilitate greater participation by persons with disabilities in the development of policy and the design and implementation of community programmes. These include:

- public education about personal choices;
- incentives to encourage greater community and consumer responsibility;
- direct consumer participation in the system such as health councils, public health boards and community health associations;
- participation in organizations that will identify needs and plan the provision of services at the community level.

CHALLENGES TO THE CURRENT SYSTEM

There are a number of community, professional and bureaucratic challenges to the current rehabilitation system. The public is demanding increased accessibility and availability of rehabilitation services. Demands for opportunities for consumer and community input in resource allocation need to be addressed. Consumers sense that a community based approach may have the potential to provide greater satisfaction than traditional institutional rehabilitation models. In addition, health professionals advocating community practice also anticipate new careers in community level rehabilitation, for example, working in education, home care, community clinics and the workplace. Community rehabilitation services may also provide an effective base for further community development in health, education, housing and employment. In this way, community services may become part of a wider decentralization and democratization of rehabilitation services.

Rehabilitation professionals have strong incentives for promoting community based services. Many professionals realize that the current structure of the rehabilitation system is not meeting consumer needs appropriately. In addition, there is an international shortage of rehabilitation professionals with a concurrent maldistribution of experienced practitioners with respect to needs of client groups, especially in rural areas. There are many political and bureaucratic interests which are now considering community services as a viable option for the delivery of rehabilitation services. These groups frequently desire to rationalize a mixture of services under one organizational entity. However, there is also a parallel desire to reduce public costs in a time of economic constraint.

The increasing costs of institutional services in all aspects of health care have led governments and agencies to develop new service delivery strategies. There is an increasing recognition that traditional hospital and physician driven systems are not necessarily the most appropriate or socially acceptable approaches. Community programmes are increasingly seen as a practical and effective alternative to conventional institutional practice. The development of community services in health and rehabilitation is a response to health resource rationalization, to changes in professional/public relationships and to an increased concern with providing effective and accessible rehabilitation programmes. The development of community services that function in collaboration with rehabilitation institutions will reduce demand on the institutional facilities which remain the most expensive part of the rehabilitation system. It is essential, however, that institutional programmes be part of the overall community strategy as institutions are not separate from the community. Until recently, both institutional and community based rehabilitation programmes have evolved independently without central planning and coordination at regional or district levels (Peat and Boyce, 1993).

THE OBJECTIVE OF COMMUNITY BASED REHABILITATION

The major objective of community based rehabilitation (CBR) is to ensure that persons with disabilities are able to maximize their physical and mental abilities, have access to regular services and opportunities and achieve full social integration within their communities and their societies (ILO, UNESCO, WHO, 1994). The principles which guide the development and implementation of CBR programmes include:

- the autonomy and dignity of individuals are respected;
- the primary responsibility for health and health care lies with the individual;
- the right to information in order to make decisions;
- the right to accept, or not to accept services;
- the right to reasonable and equitable access to rehabilitation programs (A Planning Framework, 1995).

The future development of CBR will be influenced by increased awareness among key stakeholders of what they can accomplish by working together to support community programmes which enhance equalization of opportunities and social integration for persons with disabilities. Decentralization is a key feature in the expansion of community programmes if communities are able to respond to local needs effectively. This will enhance the community's ability to have control of how rehabilitation activities can be implemented. Sustainability of programmes at the community level is only possible where the community has taken ownership of the concept and is a major stakeholder in planning, implementation and resource allocation.

FLEXIBILITY IN APPROACH

Given the diversity of communities, in terms of their structure, economy and cultures, CBR exists in many forms. There is no single blueprint for CBR, and there is no single model. Differences have to be expected because CBR will reflect the communities where it exists, and communities are different (Pupulin, 1995). Services provided by CBR are meant to enhance the current rehabilitation services structure, and are not intended to replace or duplicate existing services provided by acute and long-term care facilities. Rehabilitation services are provided along a continuum which extends from the person with a disability in the community to the specialist regional and national facility.

> **CBR is implemented through the combined efforts of disabled people themselves, their families and communities and the appropriate health, education, vocational and social services**
>
> *At the national level*, CBR should form part of a country's policy to assist all people who have any type of disability. The detailed methods of implementing CBR will vary from country to country.
>
> *At the regional and district level*, CBR should be supported with referral services and by transfer of knowledge to communities.
>
> *At the community level*, programmes should belong to the community and should be implemented under the control of the community, as represented by the local government or authority.

DEMONSTRATING THE VALUE OF COMMUNITY BASED REHABILITATION

The successful and continuing development of CBR will be influenced by the ability of its participants to demonstrate its value, cost-effectiveness and efficiency. Even if the planning of CBR is based on the recommendations of professionals, the specific demands of the consumer and the identified needs of the community, there is no assurance that the person with a disability or the community will automatically benefit. To ensure that services meet the objectives and expectations of the stakeholders, evaluation of the benefits of unique CBR strategies and services is essential. The evaluation process must be relevant and feasible and involve persons with disabilities and the community in its design and implementation. It is also essential that the community participate in the interpretation of the outcome of the evaluation process.

Research in the components of CBR is a major responsibility of all stakeholders. In a period of severe competition for limited resources, all participants share the responsibility of examining the critical factors influencing the implementation and application of CBR. Research must address:

- the magnitude of disability;
- outcome measures;
- modes of delivery;
- methods of information sharing;
- technology;
- policy;
- management.

Research findings must be widely shared and should also link CBR with other community development programmes. Research, like evaluation, must be a collaborative venture involving researchers, administrators, persons with disability and other key stakeholders. The basic objective of research is that it is relevant and contributes to the improvement of the quality of life and the integration of persons with disabilities.

The current debate on community rehabilitation services is an important element in the restructuring process currently under way in health and social systems globally. The growing awareness of fiscal limitations, consumer demands for participation in planning and operations, and a need for greater community focus should lead to an integrated system that is more accessible and committed to maintaining the person with a disability in the community.

If we could all act in a spirit of solidarity, recognizing the principles of human equality, if we could bring services to all in need, if we could contribute a better quality of life, reduce the dependency and transfer power to them, then we would restore to disabled people their right to a life in dignity. (Helander, 1994)

REFERENCES

A Planning Framework for the Community Rehabilitation Program, External Stakeholder (1995) Community Rehabilitation Working Group, Alberta Health, Alberta.

Helander, E. (1994) *Prejudice and Dignity: An Introduction to Community Based Rehabilitation.* United Nations Development Program, New York.

International Labour Organization (ILO), UNESCO, World Health Organization (WHO) (1994) *Joint Position Paper on Community Based Rehabilitation for and with People with Disabilities.* Geneva.

Jongbloed, L. and Crichton, A. (1990) A new definition of disability: implications for rehabilitation practice and social policy. *Canadian Journal of Occupational Therapy* 27: 1.

Ministry of Health Ontario (1989) Deciding the Future of Our Health Care: An overview of areas for public discussion. Toronto.

Peat, M. and Boyce, W. (1993) Canadian community rehabilitation services: challenges for the future. *Canadian Journal of Rehabilitation* 6(4): 281–289.

Pupulin, E. (1995) The concept of Community Based Rehabilitation: reflexions on current status and future perspectives. *NU News on Health Care in Developing Countries* 2/95, **9**: 4–5.

UN Statement on CBR (1995) *CBR News* No. 19, p. 5, 32–38. Appropriate Health Resources and Technologies Action Group, London.

Index

Note: CBR is used for Community Based Rehabilitation

Action Aid 105
  publications 87
Activities of Daily Living (ADL) 84
Advantages of CBR 34
Advocacy organizations 126
Age
  disability and 7–8
  of population, increasing 10–11
Aims of CBR 34–5, 156, 158
Alberta Health Insurance Plan 52
All Russia Society of the Disabled (ARSD) 123
AMREF 51
Appropriate Health Resources and
  Technologies Action Group (AHRTAG)
  83, 87
Appropriate technology 83–5
Arthritis 10
Arthritis Society of Canada 40
Arthritis Society Outreach Programme,
  Canada 66
Awareness building 119

Beneficiaries of CBR 35
Berkeley Independent Living Housing Venture
  127
Biomedical Model 6
Bosnia-Herzogovina, CBR in 44–5
Bottom-up approach 37–8
Brain injury, traumatic 10

Canadian Association of Independent Living
  Centres (CAILC) 127

Canadian Rehabilitation Council for the
  Disabled 129
Cardiac disorders 10
CARE 150
Caregivers
  as stakeholders in CBR 32
  as stakeholders in education 100
Cerebral palsy 81, 84
Charitable organizations 122
Children, preventable disability in 11–12
Coalition of Provincial Organizations of the
  Handicapped (COPOH) 123, 129
Combined Disabilities Association 25
Communication 86–7
Community
  common ties 18–19
  definition 16, 17, 18
  development, definition 22
  disadvantaged groups in 19
  entry into 21
  existing programmes 18
  governance 17–18
  historical perspective 18
  kaleidoscopic strategies 25
  leadership 17–18
  as locality 16–17
  members as stakeholders in education 100
  mobilization 23–5, 88–9
  multiplicity of 20
  participation 23–5, 88–9
    barriers to 24–5
    strengths of 23–4
  resources 17
  as social organization 17–18
  as stakeholders in CBR 33

Community based medical rehabilitation
(CBMR) 42
Community based rehabilitation 20–1
 common elements of programmes 31–2
 composition 31–4
 definition of 22, 30–1
 general principles 31
 knowledge base 98–9
 technology 82–3
 vocational rehabilitation 40, 41–2
Community Based Rehabilitation Clinics,
 Sarajevo, Bosnia-Herzegovina 69
Community Based Rehabilitation Programme,
 Scott Hospital, Morija, South Africa 53
Community Based Vocational Rehabilitation,
 Ibadan, Nigeria 67
Community initiated projects 22
Community integration program (CIP) 42
Community oriented rehabilitation 23, 38–9
Community Oriented Rehabilitation at the
 Lowenstein Hospital, Raanana, Israel 68
Community practice rehabilitation clinics,
 Canada 63
Community rehabilitation clinic 40
Community Rehabilitation Program, Alberta,
 Canada 52
Community supervisor, intermediate level,
 role of 77
Community workers 29
 role in community based rehabilitation
  programme 76–7
 as stakeholders in CBR 33
 as stakeholders in education 100
 training for 104–5
Conflict, areas of, CBR in 44–6
Consumer groups 125–6
Consumer movement 129–31
Consumer organizations 123–6
Continuum of rehabilitation 36–7
Coordination
 project 86–7
 of services 41
COPOH 123, 129
Cost-effectiveness 92
Costs 92–3
 of disability 115–18
 to the family 117–18
 to the individual with a disability 117
 loss of skill and experience 116
 measuring the implications 116–17
 to society 118

to the system 118–19
Cross-disability organizations 129

Decentralization 74
Demographics of disability 6–10
Developed countries
 disability in 10–11
 government policies in 149–50
Development of CBR, phases of 1
Disability
 definitions 4–6
 reactions to 28
Disabled Farmers of Alberta, Canada 40, 61, 81
Disabled People's International (DPI) 6, 123–5
 classification 6
Disablement, definition 6
Disadvantages of CBR 34
District Rehabilitation Centre Program, India
 80
Dom Zdravljas, Yugoslavia (house of health
 system) 40, 45

Economic environment 6, 7
Economics of disability 114–19
 see also Costs; Funding
Education 79, 99
 advanced and interdisciplinary graduate
  level 110–11
 continuing 109–10
 distance learning 109–10
 non-professional 104–7
 professional programmes 107–9
 programme design and implementation
  102–3
  core curriculum 103
  planning of courses 102–3
  site selection 102
 stakeholders in 99–101
 strategies 101–2
 through experience 104
 see also Training
Effectiveness, programme 94
Employers
 as stakeholders in CBR 33–4
 as stakeholders in education 101
Empowerment 43, 119–22
 families 121
 persons with disabilities 121–2
 professional 121
 rehabilitation systems 120

Evaluation
  models of 95–6
  participatory 95
  quantitative and qualitative 94
  use of findings 94–5
  what, how and why 90–4

Family
  in community life 19
  costs of disability 117–18
  empowerment 121
  as stakeholders in CBR 32
  as stakeholders in education 100
Fiji Disabled People's Association 129
Flexibility 158–9
Framework, descriptive, of CBR 34–6
Funding
  budget framework 81–2
  origin of programme support 80–1
Future plans 156–7

GLADNET 87
Governance 73, 92
Governments
  as stakeholders in CBR 33
  as stakeholders in education 100–1
Grassroots programmes 22
Guyana Community Based Rehabilitation
    Programme 54

Handicap, definition 4, 5
Handicapped Housing Society of Alberta 129
Health, definition of 42–3
Home Care programmes, Kingston, Canada
    40
Human rights policy 151–4

Impact, programme 93–4
Impairment, definition 4, 5, 6
Independent living movement 126–8
Infant mortality rates 7, 8
Information 79, 85, 88
Information based rehabilitation 31
Institutional services 28–9
International Classification of Disability and
    Handicap Model 6
International Classification of Impairments,
    Disabilities and Handicaps 4–6

International Labour Organization (ILO) 40,
    41–2, 87, 117, 124
Internet 87

Jaiput foot 84

Kailas Foundation, Ellora, India 40
King Edward Memorial Hospital, Bombay,
    India 39
Kingston Independent Living Resource Center
    (KILRC), Canada 60
Knowledge transfer 80, 99, 140

Leprosy 24, 28, 84, 129
Less developed countries
  disability in 11–14
  research in 142
Lifespan, increasing 10–11
Literacy 19
Local supervisors 104

Management 72–3
  of community based rehabilitation
      programmes 74–85
    programme roles and responsibilities 76–7
    strategic planning 75
    structure and organization 75–6
  functions 92
Medical model of health care and
    rehabilitation 2, 28
Mental handicaps 28
Mobility 84
Mobilization , community 88–9
Models
  aims 49
  defining and classifying 48–9
  of disablement process 6
  human resources 49
  origin 49–50
  structure 49
Multilateral agencies
  as stakeholders in CBR 33
  as stakeholders in education 100–1
Multiple sclerosis 129

National Association of the Deaf, Thailand
    129

Negros Occidental Rehabilitation Foundation (NORFI) 58
Non-government organizations (NGOs) 87
    comparison with government organizations 151
    relationships 141

Objectives of CBR 2
Organizations of persons with disabilities 122–9
Origins of CBR 28–9
Orthotic devices 84, 136
Outreach
    community 39
    network 39–40
Ownership 73

Participatory rural appraisal (PRA) 95
Performance evaluation 78
Persons United for Self-Help in Ontario (PUSH Ontario), Canada 59
Persons with a disability
    costs of disability 117
    empowerment 121
    organizations of 122–9
    as stakeholders in CBR 32
    as stakeholders in education 99–100
Physical environment 6, 7
Physically Challenged Farmers of Alberta, Canada 61
Planning 72–3
Policies 79
    analysis 141
    government 149–50
    human rights 151–4
    making 143–4
    multilateral agencies and governmental collaborative 150–1
    non-government organization 150
    public 89, 146–9
        CBR and policy development 148–9
        factors influencing development 147–8
        identification of 148
        public participation in development of 144–6
        strategic planning and development of 146–9
Poliomyelitis 10, 81, 84, 100
Poverty 9–10, 19
Pragathi Creations, Bangalore, India 81

Prevalence of disability, global estimates 12–14
Professional rehabilitation personnel
    empowerment 121
    role in community based rehabilitation programme 77–8
    as stakeholders in CBR 33
    as stakeholders in education 101
PROJIMO 70
Prosthetic devices 84, 136
Pulmonary disorders 10

Quality of Life Model 6

Rayalaseema Sava Samithi (RASS) 56
Recruitment 93
Rehabilitation
    challenges to current system 157–8
    definition 1–2
Rehabilitation skill transfer 80
Relevance of evaluation of CBR 93
Reporting mechanisms of disability 8–9
Research, rehabilitation
    difficulties in 137–8
    funding limitations 138
    goal of 137–8
    interest in 137
    in less developed countries 142
    partnerships in 141–2
    topics 138–41
Resources
    allocation of 43–4
    human 93
    local 79
    local structures 79
    physical 78–9
    supporting CBR programmes 35–6
Rural areas, rehabilitation resources in 11

Sahaya CBR Project, India 56
Save the Children 150
Self-advocacy 126
Self-help organizations 129
Self-organizing 119
Seva-in-Action Production and Training Centre, Bangalore, India 81
Silent World Craft, Bangkok, Thailand 81
Skill transfer 99, 140
Social environment 6, 7

Soft tissue injuries 10
SOURABHA CBR Programme for the
    Disabled, India 57, 105
Spinal cord injury 10
Sri Lanka Federation of the Visually
    Handicapped 129
Stakeholders
    in CBR 32
    in education 99–101
Strategies
    of CBR 35, 37–8
    for changes toward CBR 42–3
    in education 101–2
Stroke 10, 84
Support advocacy 126
Sustainability, programme 85–6
'Sveti Duh' hospital, Zagreb, Croatia 39
Swedish Deaf Project 129
System advocacy 126

Terry Fox Mobile Clinic 65
Top-down approach 37–8
Trainers
    role in community based rehabilitation
        programme 76
Training 44, 79, 93
    community vocational training programmes
        40
    for community workers 104–7
    non-professional 104–7
    organization of 103
    potential problems 103–4
    for teachers of teachers 107
    see also Education
Training manuals 29–30
Trauma 10
Travelling Clinics of Newfoundland and
    Labrador, Children's rehabilitation
    center 64
Tuberculosis 10, 28
Types of disabilities 14

Uni-disability organizations 129
UNICEF 29

Union of Palestinian Medical Relief
    Committees (UPMRC) 55
United Nations
    Economic and Social Council Organization
        124
    International Decade of Disabled Persons
        29, 105, 151
    International Year of Disabled Persons 151
    Standard Rules of Equalization of
        Opportunities for Persons with
        Disabilities 151–4
    World Program of Action Concerning
        Disabled Persons 131, 151
University of Eindhoven, Netherlands, Faculty
    of Appropriate Technology 83
Urban areas, rehabilitation resources in 11

Value of CBR 159–60
Village health workers 104
Voluntarism 24
Voluntary Health Services Society (VHSS),
    Bangladesh 80
Volunteers
    role in community based rehabilitation
        programme 77
    as stakeholders in CBR 33
    as stakeholders in education 100

Women, role of 88, 131–2, 140
World Bank 100
World Blind Union 150
World Federation of the Deaf 150
World Health Assembly (1976) 29
World Health Organization 28, 29, 124
    Health for All 74
World Institute on Disability (WID) 125
World Program of Action Concerning Disabled
    Persons 124
World-wide web 87

Yee Hong Community Wellness Foundation,
    Scarborough, Canada 62